REFORM AND REGULATION IN LONG-TERM CARE

REFORM AND REGULATION IN LONG-TERM CARE

Edited by

Valerie La Porte
Jeffrey Rubin

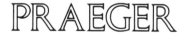

PRAEGER

PRAEGER SPECIAL STUDIES • PRAEGER SCIENTIFIC

Library of Congress Cataloging in Publication Data

Main entry under title:

Reform and regulation in long-term care.

Includes index.
   1. Long-term care of the sick--United States.
2. Long-term care of the sick--United States--Finance.
3. Nursing homes--United States.   I. LaPorte, Valerie.
II. Rubin, Jeffrey, 1949-
RA644.6.R44   362.1'6'0973   79-9761
ISBN 0-03-049341-2

Portions of this study were funded by the Office of
the Assistant Secretary for Planning and Evaluation,
Office of Social Services and Human Development, Department
of Health, Education and Welfare. Any opinions, findings,
conclusions, or recommendations expressed are those of
the author(s) and do not necessarily reflect the view of
the Department of Health, Education and Welfare.

PRAEGER PUBLISHERS, PRAEGER SPECIAL STUDIES
383 Madison Avenue, New York, N.Y. 10017, U.S.A.

Published in the United States of America in 1979
by Praeger Publishers,
A Division of Holt, Rinehart and Winston, CBS, Inc.

9   038   987654321

Printed in the United States of America

PREFACE

The size of the long-term care population and the magnitude of resources devoted to this group provide a clear justification for this volume. In a recent estimate, the Congressional Budget Office placed the population in need of long-term care in 1975 between 5.5 and 9.9 million people.[1] The same office also estimated that the array of public programs that finance long-term care services spent $5.7 billion in 1975. Medicaid provided the bulk of these funds, allocating most of its $4.4 billion to nursing home care. Private sources paid out an additional $5.9 to $7.7 billion; almost 90 percent of this sum consisted of out-of-pocket expenditures by individuals. Long-term care also poses substantial indirect costs for individuals and the economy in general in the form of foregone productivity.

The facts and figures alone could probably not account for the emerging interest in long-term care. Recently, however, observers have pointed to serious deficiences in the system of care for the chronically ill and impaired, and many members of the public are beginning to question the performance of government and the health industry in this area. First, there is evidence that between 800,000 and 1,400,000 people are presently in need of long-term care but do not receive any services. Second, much of the care provided in nursing homes and community facilities has been judged to be inadequate. Third, the system of long-term care in the United States appears to be biased toward institutional forms of care, leading to the placement of individuals in facilities unsuited to their specific needs. Finally, as the population distribution shifts toward the upper age brackets, a higher proportion of the population can be expected to stand in need of long-term care services. In fact, the Congressional Budget Office estimates that the potential population needing long-term care services will grow from between 5.5 and 9.9 million in 1975 to between 7.4 and 12.5 million in 1985. Thus, the task of providing adequate services, in appropriate settings, to all individuals who have need of them will in all likelihood become more difficult in the years ahead.

It was in recognition of these problems and in the hope that solutions could be found that the Office of Social Services and Human Development in the Department of Health, Education, and Welfare commissioned the four overview chapters which form the core of this volume. Subsequently, in order to extend its study of the long-term care system in the United States, the Office joined with Rutgers University to sponsor a seminar which would pursue the discussion of particular policy questions. This anthology brings together the original studies, each a comprehensive treatment of a long-term care issue and its background, and the briefer position papers and commentaries which were presented at the seminar in January 1978. In compiling a somewhat heterogeneous collection of this kind, we have sought to reproduce the variety of approaches and opinions that the authors and seminar participants brought to the subject of long-term care. We have also sought to recapture in the volume the spirit of dialogue and productive exchange that prevailed at the seminar.

The authors represent several different disciplines, and their papers touch upon very different elements of the system: the design of service programs, the financing of long-term care, the monitoring of facilities and programs by government regulatory agencies and auditors, and the cost impact of regulation upon the provider and the economy in general. The wide range of subjects not only reflects the different professional backgrounds of the contributors to the volume, but also attests to the fact that policy questions in the field of long-term care do not admit any one-sided solutions. What emerges very distinctly in a review of the volume is that collaboration among government agencies, legislators, and program administrators will be necessary before any significant imrpovements in the system of long-term care can be made.

NOTE

1. U.S., Congress, Congressional Budget Office, *Long Term Care for the Elderly and Disabled*, by Maureen S. Baltay, Budget Issue Paper, February 1977 (Washington, D.C.: Government Printing Office), Table 3, p. 8. This figure does not include the nearly 200,000 persons in state and county psychiatric hospitals, as well as those persons in other long-term pychiatric facilities.

All subsequent statistics on the long-term care population and program expenditures in this and the following paragraph are drawn from the Budget Paper, pp. 8–16.

ACKNOWLEDGMENTS

We wish to thank the authors and seminar participants who contributed to this volume. It is their experience, effort, and insight which are represented in the pages of this volume, and the book is, in substance, their own.

We wish to acknowledge also the assistance of John Noble and John De Wilde of the Department of Health, Education, and Welfare. Their concern for identifying solutions to the problems in the long-term care sector led to the undertaking of this project. Monroe Berkowitz, Director of the Disability and Health Economic Research Section of the Bureau of Economic Research at Rutgers University, planned the seminar on issues in long-term care and selected the papers for presentation. Stephen McConnell shared in the editing chores, and Laura Ford and Lynne Lavigne helped to prepare the manuscript.

CONTENTS

LIST OF TABLES

REFORM AND REGULATION IN LONG-TERM CARE

1
INTRODUCTION

Valerie LaPorte
Jeffrey Rubin

THE LONG-TERM CARE POPULATION
AND PUBLIC PROGRAMS

The field of long-term care poses several fundamental problems for public policy. The first is that of defining the population in question: who makes up the "long-term care population"? The name itself implies that the characteristic that unites the members of this group is the chronic nature of their condition. But the duration of an illness or impairment is not the only factor that determines the need for long-term care services. Rather, the individuals who are conventionally included in this group—the aged, the mentally ill, and the physically and developmentally disabled— have a chronic condition that combines with other personal characteristics to render them incapable of performing one or more normal daily activities. It is this inability to carry out certain routine tasks that is the distinguishing feature of the long-term care population.

There is clearly a great deal of overlap between the long-term care population and the disabled. The degree to which the two groups intersect becomes evident if we consider the definition of disability offered in much of the recent literature on the subject. The disabled individual is identified as one unable to perform a socially expected role because of the combined effect of a physical or mental impairment with personal and environmental factors. If we were to push the definition of the long-term care population and the definition of the disabled to their extremes, the two would seem to merge. In actuality, however, the definitions usually have more restricted applications. Disability describes an individual's inability to function in such major life roles as work, housework, and education; long-term care suggests an individual's inability to perform the activities necessary to daily living, such as cooking, bathing, or getting about the home.

The distinction between the two groups can be further clarified by considering the kinds of services associated with the long-term care population and the disabled. Members of both groups may be in need of medical services. But individuals who are candidates for long-term care services most often have a medical condition that has stabilized. They rarely require intensive physician care, and some form of medical maintenance is typical of the health care they receive. More important for the long-term care population are personal care, social, and support services. These services are designed to provide the members of this population with assistance in carrying out normal daily activities.

Services for the disabled, on the other hand, are intended to restore the individual to a productive vocational role. The emphasis in services for the disabled is on rehabilitation, and the objective is the return of the individual to work or homemaking activities.

A second policy issue concerns the nature of, and rationale for, government intervention in the area of long-term care. The long-term care population is eligible for transfer payments under a number of federal programs. Individuals with a record of work experience who become disabled after attaining an insured status are eligible for Social Security Disability Insurance benefits. Workers who are injured on the job and who give up their right to sue their employer in a tort claim are entitled to workers' compensation benefits. Disabled veterans receive benefits if they have established a period of military service, and for those who demonstrate need by a means test, the Supplemental Security Income program offers assistance in the form of transfer payments.

In addition to providing cash transfers, federal programs also make certain services available to the long-term care population. Medicaid, Medicare, and the state-federal vocational rehabilitation program are the principal programs that finance medical care and rehabilitation services. Housing and transportation services are offered under other state and federal programs.

The public programs are clearly designed to compensate for the losses experienced by individuals with chronic disease and disability. Some programs are intended to relieve the physical, mental, and psychological ill effects of disability, others, to make up for the loss of wage earning capacity. Critics point out, however, that the programs that were created as "the solution" to the problems of the long-term care population may have given rise to a new set of difficulties. For example, the provision of health services is in itself necessary and beneficial. But if the services are tied to a set of restrictive conditions—narrowly defined eligibility criteria or limitations on the duration of benefits—then some members of the long-term care population may not be able to take advantage of them. In this case, a restructuring of existing programs might be necessary to accommodate those persons who require health services on a continuing and perhaps indefinite basis.

Regulation is another form of government intervention that may have unanticipated consequences. Regulation is undertaken to protect the interests of the public and to prevent abuses in the health industry. There is some evidence, however, that the costs of regulation are not sufficiently understood. Nursing home administrators charge that compliance with new regulations places unrealistic financial demands upon them; researchers contend that the macroeconomic consequences of regulation deserve further study and should be considered before regulations are promulgated.

What the extent of government involvement in the area of long-term care should be, and what forms that involvement should take, are matters open to dispute. Several of the authors in this volume address these questions, and in many of their policy recommendations, they suggest a role for the government which would make intervention a positive force.

PERSPECTIVES ON LONG-TERM CARE: THE AUTHORS

The authors whose work is represented in this volume undertook to examine the problems of the long-term care system and to recommend certain directions for policy reform. The picture of the system that emerges from their accounts is a troubling one: care is inadequate yet costly; the delivery of services, uncertain; and the mechanisms for financing care, inefficient or discriminatory. Institutional care continues to be the prevalent form of care, despite the disclosures in recent years of inadequate care and improper management practices in some nursing homes and mental health institutions. While the growing consensus among professionals is that institutions may be an undesirable and needlessly restrictive setting for many members of the chronically ill and impaired population, government efforts to develop alternative long-term care facilities have been fairly limited to date. Those individuals whose needs might best be served in a home setting or in small residential facilities closely integrated with the community are often inappropriately placed because community services of this type are scarce and poorly funded.

There is agreement among the authors that serious "structural barriers" to the efficient provision of services also exist. Because the long-term care population is a somewhat heterogeneous group, a variety of agencies administer to their health, social, and economic needs. A failure to cooperate on the part of these agencies means that individual clients may not receive the necessary "stream" of services, and variations in program eligibility criteria may mean that certain clients are overlooked altogether. Several authors also stress the inequities of the system. The states have failed to provide a uniform level of care; allocations for long-term care differ from state to state, and discrepancies in the quality and range of services have emerged. Finally, the authors point to the conceptual misunderstanding that surrounds the notion of "long-term care." Policymakers continue to regard long-term care as health care; they fail to acknowledge that the medical needs of this population have stabilized to the point where only some form of medical management is necessary. As a consequence of this error, policymakers have minimized the importance of the social and psychological needs of the population.

While the authors are fairly consistent in their analyses of the system's shortcomings, they differ as to the best means of remedying the problems. There are a number of avenues open to policymakers who hope to improve long-term care services. Reforms can be carried out at the level of the services themselves; changes can be made in the types of services offered, the settings in which services are made available, and the methods for coordinating services and overseeing the progress of individual clients. While the redesign of service programs is perhaps the most direct approach to the problem of long-term care, other opportunities for policy reform do exist. The financing of long-term care presents one such opportunity. Changes in the administration of public funds under the Medicaid program would clearly have repercussions at the service level. Certain of the authors represented in this volume urge that federal monies should be redirected to service providers and populations neglected by Medicaid at present; in this way, the redistribution of funds could itself become a means of realizing a new set of long-term care priorities. Other authors call for the reexamination of the roles of state and federal governments in the financing of long-term care and question whether the states' discretionary powers should be expanded or reduced.

Change can also be brought about by the monitoring of the long-term care system. Government regulation of skilled nursing facilities and intermediate care facilities, audit investigations of these same facilities, and the involvement of the courts in the operation of institutions all represent possibilities for evaluating and improving the performance of the long-term care system.

THE OVERVIEW PAPERS

As we indicated above, the papers in this volume have different origins. The comprehensive overview papers contracted for by the Office of Social Services and Human Development make up Chapters 2–5 of the volume; Chapters 6–9 represent the contribution of the participants to the long-term care seminar. We begin our survey of papers and the policy recommendations they contain with a brief consideration of "Long-Term Care: A Challenge to Service Systems," the second of the overview papers.

In the opening chapter of the volume, Judith LaVor directs her attention to the design and delivery of services for the long-term care population. Contending that the lack of interprogram coordination poses difficulties for all members of this population, the author presents a framework for an organized *system* of long-term care. The system comprises a range of health, social, and economic services and includes as its most prominent feature a mechanism for coordinating services at the client level. While the coordination mechanism could, theoretically, take a number of forms, a specific model is presented in the proposal for an "Ambulatory Chronic Care Service" (ACCS), which concludes the chapter. Here LaVor calls for the creation of local agencies that would evaluate client needs, prescribe services, and monitor client progress. The contention underlying the entire argument is that service structures should be made flexible enough to accommodate the individual's particular combination of needs by providing the client with an appropriate package of services and supports.

LaVor's proposed solutions are oriented less toward major program reform than toward the adaptation and coordination of existing resources. She recommends, for example, the possibility of an exchange or integration of comunity and institutional services and the possibility of realigning programs so that the same providers and service mechanisms might serve people whose conditions or required levels of care differ. While the ACCS proposal necessitates the creation of a new agency at the community level, this agency is essentially a kind of liaison, designed to oversee and coordinate the operations of existing programs and service providers.

In the third chapter of this volume, Edward Correia sets forth a more ambitious program of reform. Directing his attention to the financing of long-term care, he calls for the actual restructuring of the Medicaid system, presently the principal channel for public long-term care funds. Correia's concerns in this chapter stem from his dissatisfaction with the provisions made for the chronically ill and disabled under the various proposals for national health insurance. While the majority of the proposals call for the dissolution of a comprehensive Medicaid program, many would retain Medicaid financing in the area of long-term care. These proposals, Correia argues, would only perpetuate the high costs, poor standards, and limited access to care which are associated with Medicaid at present. While Correia recognizes that a national health insurance program in some form is a likely eventuality, his belief that existing proposals do not come to terms with the needs of the long-term care population leads him to offer his own model for the financing of long-term care. The model involves a redistribution of the powers of the federal and state governments in the area of long-term care. The federal government would be responsible for the institutional component of the program, guaranteeing every person access to skilled nursing facilities (SNFs) and intermediate care facilities (ICFs). While the federal government now oversees the state-administered individual entitlement programs for SNF and ICF care, its control over these programs would be extended. As Correia envisions its role, the federal government would ensure that eligibility requirements, cost-sharing requirements, and quality standards were uniform in every state. The states, on the other hand, would assume greater responsibility in the administration of funds for noninstitutional services. They would have at their disposal expanded federal grants for these services and could allocate the grant funds as they saw fit. Correia suggests that the states are more sensitive to local needs than the federal government, and are, therefore, better suited to choose those health, social, and support services that should be made available to their resident populations. The states, moreover, can be relied upon to take the initiative in developing such alternatives to institutional care as day care, home health, and congregate care.

In the fourth chapter in this volume Hirsch Ruchlin examines government intervention in the long-term health care industry, paying particular attention to the role of the federal and state agencies in the regulation of nursing homes. Ruchlin argues that regulation has been largely ineffective in achieving its goals—the improvement of industry performance and the insurance of a socially acceptable level of care—and he attempts to identify the problems that have undermined the effectiveness of regulatory programs. One of the author's principal findings is that government constraints may have failed to produce the desired industry behavior because they have not given sufficient weight to the economic self-interest of the provider. His analysis leads him to argue for a reform of the incentive structure in the health industry, and, in particular, the introduction of a procedure for recompensing the providers of high quality care.

The first stage in this procedure is an inspection of long-term care facilities, directed toward considerations of patient welfare. Each facility would be assigned a "patient health status index" as a measure of its performance in meeting the medical and psychosocial needs of its patients. Regulatory agencies might then adjust the reimbursement rate for each SNF or ICF in accordance with the facility index. Those facilities which rendered a high level of care would be reimbursed at a higher rate. In this way, Ruchlin's scheme would accommodate the economic self-interest of the provider and create the necessary incentives to improve patient environment and care.

Regulation is only one method of monitoring the long-term care system which might prove instrumental in the improvement of services. In the fifth chapter of this volume, Robert M. Dias examines a second method, the auditing of long-term care and disability programs. Dias argues that the audit function has been misunderstood by policymakers and legislators and that its usefulness as a management tool has gone unrecognized. So that government groups and program personnel might take fuller advantage of the audit program in general, as well as the findings of particular investigations, Dias offers several recommendations for audit reform.

Foremost among the changes that Dias suggests is the expansion of the role of audit. Audit could become an effective means of achieving improved program accountability. State audit agencies might undertake routine "program" or "performance" audits in addition to monitoring the fiscal operations of the long-term care and disability programs. The agencies would not only examine the financial transactions and accounts of the programs, but would also seek to determine whether management had been successful in achieving its program objectives. So that audit findings might have a greater impact on program policy and management practices, Dias outlines specific follow-up measures. These measures are designed to ensure that program officials take action to correct deficiencies reported by the auditors and to implement the recommendations of the auditors. Throughout his discussion of the audit function, Dias stresses the contributions that audit can make to program management. He cautions against the tendency of policymakers to conceive of auditing as an activity entirely independent of the effective functioning of long-term care and disability programs.

In addition to reconsidering the relationship of audit and program management, Dias suggests certain changes in the internal organization of audit groups. Specifically, he calls for the creation of a single audit program at the state level that would assume the responsibilities now shared by different government groups. Dias contends that substituting a comprehensive audit program for the present multiple agency system would eliminate problems of duplicate coverage and bring about a more efficient use of resources.

THE SEMINAR PAPERS

In his paper Thomas Walsh presents a detailed analysis of a cost-related reimbursement model for long-term care facilities. The analysis is based upon Walsh's own experience in establishing such a system in Illinois. The method incorporates the cost differentials associated with caring for patients with unequal needs. Recognizing the way the long-term care market functions, Walsh identifies several of the problems likely to occur when reimbursement is too high, too low, or undifferentiated by patient.

Although an advocate of the point system, Walsh does not fail to consider some of the problems associated with patient-related reimbursement. Administrative difficulty, incomplete accounting for all needs, and the difficulty of accurately relating need to cost are cited as areas of concern.

The author then moves on to a consideration of how best to adjust costs to patient needs. Two methodologies, statistical and engineering, are examined. The statistical model is empirically estimated and judged to be of greater value. The findings of the estimated cost function in the statistical model confirm the hypothesized relationships between cost and patient needs and level of care.

The issue of government regulation of nursing homes is considered by Harvey Wertlieb. As an administrator of a nursing home, Wertlieb approaches this issue with an understanding of its import and consequences for the regulated facility. His views differ significantly from those of the academic or the policymaker, and his statement offers an illuminating contrast to the other papers included in this volume.

Wertlieb traces the irregular growth of the nursing home industry, emphasizing the economic and financial constraints leading to inadequate facilities. In addition, he shows how the intervention of the federal government does not solve existing problems but in fact creates new problems.

It is Wertlieb's contention that much of the recent criticism of nursing home facilities has been misplaced and that the fault does not lie exclusively with the provider. He cites professional disregard of the geriatric field and regulatory inflexibility as two major hindrances to the improved performance of the long-term care facility that are often overlooked by the critics of the industry. He suggests further that the public lacks a clear understanding of the extent of the problems of the aged and the handicapped and has not committed itself fully to meet the needs of these groups. Wertlieb would have us recognize that the provision of services in the long-term care facility is only one part in a system designed to help the disadvantaged cope with their problems. The long-term care facility can provide higher quality care, as well as an expanded program of services, but it cannot bring about these changes without the cooperation of the government and the public.

The author concludes by calling for recognition of the limitations of regulation and of the problems—particularly financial problems—that long-term care facilities encounter in their efforts to comply with federal regulations. A series of recommendations, largely designed to help attain the goals of regulation without the corresponding inequities, are included.

Harvey Carmel presents the results of an effort to develop and test a model designed to measure the complete cost impact of long-term care regulations. The paper begins with a review of the factors likely to influence the level of nursing home costs. Carmel shows that total operating costs can be attributed to 13 cost centers, with nursing and dietary services accounting for over 50 percent of the costs in the sample. The identification of these cost centers is the necessary first step in the construction of the model.

Relating a particular regulation to the affected cost centers is a difficult task. Carmel elaborates upon two problems of special concern: the assessment of second order effects and the interpretation of vaguely worded regulations.

The model Carmel describes is applied to facilities in Minnesota at their November 1975 status. The findings indicate that cost increases associated with coming into full compliance with existing regulations would add 3 to 10 percent to average annual facility expenditures. Carmel points to the distributional impact of these increases, contending that federal regulations affect not only federal health care programs but private insurers and individuals as well. Carmel also summarizes the varying effects of regulations with respect to cost centers and institutional characteristics such as location and ownership.

The Carmel study shows both the feasibility and necessity of reviewing regulations for their impact on long-term care costs. The influence of regulations on costs highlights the need to relate reimbursement to regulatory policy. Further linkages of regulations to patient assessment are also suggested. Finally, Carmel gives some attention to the need for improved data collection systems in long-term care institutions.

AREAS OF AGREEMENT

While the solutions posed by the authors focus on different aspects of the long-term care system, certain areas of agreement exist. LaVor, Ruchlin, and Correia are alike in urging a departure from the "medical model" of long-term care. They indicate that the greater part of public expenditures in the field of long-term care are directed toward health services, despite the growing recognition that the medical needs of most members of the population in question are limited. In particular, the authors point to the Medicaid program as being largely responsible for the perpetuation of the medical model. The first area of agreement that emerges, then, is the need for a very fundamental change in our conceptions of long-term care. LaVor, for example, recommends that we replace our present "sickness-oriented system" of long-term care with a multidimensional program combining health, social, and economic services, and that we place greater emphasis on the development of social and support services in the home and community. Ruchlin, concentrating on the narrower field of nursing homes, describes the ideal setting for long-term care as a residential and social facility with medical support provided only as necessary. The consensus is that public programs should be reoriented toward support and psychosocial services.

Several authors agree also on the necessity of making significant changes in the Medicaid program. Ruchlin and Correia would federalize Medicaid so as to eliminate the "double jeopardy" problem associated with the matching funds principle. Institutional care would be put entirely under federal control in order to insure conformity of expenditures and to promote equality of care in all states. The authors also seek an end to the Medicaid bias toward institutional care. Because federal reimbursement under this program is largely tied to services rendered in intermediate care and skilled nursing facilities, the states are encouraged to rely heavily on institutional forms of care to meet the needs of their chronically ill and impaired residents. Thus, the authors recommend that the reimbursement policy under Medicaid be changed so that less intensive forms of care in a home or community setting would be covered.

The reform of Medicaid described involves, in a sense, the substitution of an incentive toward community care for the present incentive toward institutional care. Several of the authors see the creation of new incentives and the manipulation of economic interests as the key to bringing about more appropriate or higher quality care. Ruchlin maintains that at the present time providers have little incentive to upgrade patient environment or services. However, if each facility were evaluated on the basis of its actual effectiveness in promoting patient welfare, and if its reimbursement rates were adjusted accordingly, then the profit factor might induce providers to upgrade the quality of life and services offered in their facilities.

Just as Ruchlin would use regulatory measures to motivate providers to improve institutional facilities, so Correia would adopt certain financing measures as a spur to state action in the development of community services. The financial incentives that he proposes would have a significant effect on the states' position. At present, as we have seen, it is not in the states' interest to fund services outside of the SNF or ICF setting. Correia recommends that expanded grants be made available to the states specifically for the purpose of building a noninstitutional program of services. Grants for these services would be made on a 60 percent federal-40 percent state basis, a ratio which would in itself encourage state investment in this area. Another aspect of Correia's program, a cost-sharing arrangement for institutional care, would discourage inappropriate recourse to institutional care.

The authors concur also on the need for improved coordination of the programs serving the long-term care population and of the agencies which in turn monitor the programs. The division of responsibility in the areas of regulation and auditing may mean that the findings of inspection teams or investigative groups are neglected and their recommendations unenforced. As a means of strengthening the present regulatory efforts, Ruchlin proposes that the activities of inspection and rate-setting be carried out by one agency. In this way, a facility's performance, as judged by the inspectors, would be taken into account in establishing its rate of reimbursement. Dias calls for closer cooperation between audit groups and program administrators. Management and audit teams would both participate in certain follow-up procedures to ensure that deficiencies reported by auditors were corrected and recommendations followed. Moreover, management could look to audit for assistance in determining whether particular programs had achieved their objectives. This measure would entail expanding the role of audit to include the "program" or "performance" review described earlier. Finally, Dias calls for the consolidation of the audit role within one group at the state level. At present, the Health, Education, and Welfare Audit Agency, the U.S. General Accounting Office, and state auditors frequently conduct audits of the same operations and derive similar findings; given the limited resources available for audit, some kind of merger is necessary.

LaVor works a third variation on the theme of interprogram coordination. She cites the fact that public programs are characterized by the separation of health from social and economic services. The Medicaid and Social Service programs, for example, do not "mesh"; their eligibility criteria differ. LaVor argues that the split in services could be most easily remedied at the client level. Her proposal for a community agency to oversee the progress of individual clients, making sure that each received that combination of services he or she needed, is her solution to the problem of program discontinuity.

The adoption of a social health model of long-term care, the reform of Medicaid, and the creation of incentives to state action in the field of noninstitutional services are all related to yet another policy objective that most of the authors uphold. This is the need for expansion of community care services: day care, home health care, transportation services, homemaker services, counseling, and so forth. Many of the authors suggest that services rendered in the community or home setting are the most appropriate and possibly the least costly means of caring for a large segment of the long-term care population.

POLICY CHANGE AND THE LONG-TERM SECTOR

So far in these introductory comments we have examined the basic nature of the long-term sector, the current and future need for these services, and the general areas of agreement in policy matters among the authors. It is now appropriate that we consider the difficulties which policymakers might encounter in implementing the various reforms suggested for the long-term care sector.

Many of the policy suggestions in this report were conceived as a means of bringing about two very basic changes: the improvement of institutional care and the expansion of community care. Several authors call for the transfer of some part of our present long-term care resources from institutional to noninstitutional services on the grounds that this step would promote a higher level of care and a more flexible program of services. It is an argument that commands almost immediate assent; the commitment to community and home care reflects a forward-looking attitude toward human services and would seem to be fairly easy to put into effect. Nevertheless, such a commitment might be more problematic than it at first appears.

Efforts to reduce the number or size of institutional facilities will encounter opposition from different quarters and may give rise to a new set of difficulties. We might begin our consideration of these difficulties by asking why institutions have survived the criticism to which they have been subjected at earlier periods in time. Foremost among the explanations usually offered for the durability of the institution is the simple fact that it is the type of environment in which services can be delivered most efficiently. When people having relatively similar needs are housed together, substantial economies are possible. It is easier and cheaper to feed 50 people in one building than to meet the needs of these same individuals in a variety of independent settings. The same reasoning applies to the delivery of most other services.

A second fact accounting for the continued presence of institutions is the high cost of moving people out of institutions. Even though a methodologically sound benefit-cost analysis of deinstitutionalization might show positive results, there is a great probability that some of those bearing the costs will receive few, if any, benefits. Some people will lose jobs, others will lose profitable businesses, and some persons and governmental agencies will bear a portion of the community cost. Perhaps those who would suffer a net loss as a result of the closing or reduction in size of an institution are in a minority; still, their opposition, if vocalized, might create strong political pressure against such a policy change.

The political framework in which policy options are considered must always be acknowledged. This is particularly so in the case of long-term care, where those in favor of maintaining institutions are in a stronger position than those academics and social service workers who favor community care. Another potential source of support for the deinstitutionalization movement, the institutionalized population itself, is not yet a major political force. The simple presence of many of these people in long-term care facilities attests to their powerlessness. Many of them are placed in these facilities not as a result of their own decisions but because of the decision of others.

The last argument carries within it the seeds of another justification for the continued existence of institutions. Some people do choose to enter an institution voluntarily; for others, institutionalization is simply a necessity. In both cases, the attraction of the institution may be the same: it offers a comprehensive set of services. In the well-run institution, all of a person's needs can be met and the difficulties of living alone or with family avoided.

All of these arguments are, of course, subject to discussion and debate. There are those who believe that institutions are inherently bad and that no quality care can be provided in such a setting. It is clear, however, that a significant number of people perceive a continuing need for institutions. The task, then, will be one of improving existing institutions, as well as easing the economic, political, and "tactical" complications of a shift toward community care.

To accomplish the first objective, policymakers need only look at the past performance of institutions. Evidence shows that some institutions work and work well. Improvement of existing facilities can be undertaken if we learn why certain institutions function effectively. The second objective, that of facilitating a shift toward community care, would necessitate a number of changes. The greater reliance on small group residences or homes within the community to house the chronically ill and impaired may make for a less efficient provision of care than is possible in the institution. Specific improvements in technology and transportation should be considered in devising methods of compensating for some of the inefficiencies. Innovative plans to make bulk purchases or to bring patients in need of therapy together would go a long way in reducing this particular advantage institutions have over community long-term care.

Policymakers who encourage a shift toward community care would also do well to take the entire picture into view. If workers are likely to lose jobs, if some businesses are likely to lose money, and if some families might be inconvenienced, plans must be developed to generate the support of these persons. Without at least some type of tacit support, obtacles to a changeover will surely arise. Governments are often large enough to absorb some workers if they cannot be retrained for community care. Fair offers of compensation or some alternative purchase arrangement could be made if businesses dependent on an institution are endangered by plans to convert to a community care network for long-term care.

Perhaps the most significant factor governing the success of efforts to improve institutions and to expand community care is the level of political support for such actions. Minimal or weak approval of these objectives will surely leave any legislative effort to allocate more resources to long-term care at the mercy of its critics. Only when broad support is generated can we expect sufficient resources to follow. This type of support is necessary because the public must possess a level of willingness to help those in need of long-term care before legislators will attempt to use tax revenues to upgrade institutions and initiate new community programs.

There are numerous variables that will influence the public's desire and willingness to expand publicly supported long-term care programs. Much as with the demand for other public services such as schools and fire and police protection, economic factors must be considered. Thus, the price of long-term care, the level of public income, the price of alternatives to institutionalization, and the demands for other public services (which in turn affects the overall tax rate) can all influence the public's support for improvements in long-term care.

But while each of these variables may have a role to play, a more fundamental determinant of political support exists. We have in mind what is referred to as tastes or preferences or values. The stronger the individual's attachment to a particular objective (holding the other variables constant), the more likely he will be to support, both politically and economically, its attainment. While the question of how values or preferences are formed is a matter for students of human nature, it is of concern to us that such preferences exist and that they constrain, in some significant way, political and economic support for changes in the delivery of long-term care. We would surely expect a person who places great value on all individuals' right to liberty and health to support recommendations to improve the quality of institutions and expand community facilities.

While our arguments and observations in this section of the introduction might strike the reader as cautious, or even conservative, in temper, our intention has simply been to underscore the difficulty of bringing about change in the long-term care sector and to point up the ramifications of change. We do not discourage reform; rather we seek to establish the complex economic and political framework within which reforms must be carried out. It is important to identify those changes in the areas of program design, regulation, financing, and audit that would lead to an improved level of care for the long-term care population. The authors included in this volume are engaged in exactly this task. Nevertheless, we cannot simply will these changes into effect. Efforts should be directed toward securing greater support by presenting the case of those in need of long-term care. People must be convinced of the value of such care, the rights of the long-term care population, and the necessity of providing better long-term care. The extent to which this process should occur in the political forum, the media, or the courts is an open question. All these mechanisms have been used; sometimes meeting with success, at other times, with failure. But those who advocate changes in long-term care should continue to make their case to a broad audience. The public must be convinced of the need for long-term care services and show its willingness to commit the necessary resources.

We hope this introductory discussion has put the chapters that follow into perspective for the readers. The authors vary in their support of particular changes, but each focuses to some degree on means to improve long-term care. Whatever the suggested change, be it better control and regulation of publicly spent money or a newly organized system for delivering community care, the proponents of that change must be cognizant of the political, legal, and economic realities. As these realities change, either through direct attempts at manipulation or more slowly by the impact of the normal course of events, policy analysts must be ready with proposals to meet the public's increased willingness to support improvement in the delivery of long-term care.

2
LONG-TERM CARE: A CHALLENGE TO SERVICE SYSTEMS

Judith LaVor

THE LONG-TERM CARE POPULATION AND ITS SERVICE NEEDS: AN INTRODUCTION

The phrase "long-term care" describes services for the chronically ill and the physically and mentally disabled whose conditions are not amenable to brief periods of treatment. The difficulties of financing the multiple services required by this clientele have, of course, been widely acknowledged. But while the fame, or infamy, of long-term care grows with each billion dollars added to the bill for institutional care, more significant issues than the control of cost should command the attention of the public and the government. Those issues represent one of the most interesting challenges in the human services field today: how can the plethora of health, social, and income services currently offered under a number of independent programs be organized to provide care and service to populations whose needs do not fall into a single neat category?

The successful organization and delivery of services to this group could be the starting point for a reevaluation of the human services system in the United States. The goal may seem elusive, in part because care of the chronically ill and impaired still has a low status in the medical and health professions. But this system is for the first time being forced, in the area of chronic illness and disability, to deal with a combination of services and to look at the client as a multidimensioned being with a variety of medical, economic, and social needs. We are now faced with the need to make our

The author wishes to thank Marie Callender and Brahna Trager, who shared in the development of the ideas presented in this chapter.

category-oriented system work to the benefit of the consumer with multiple needs. Coordination, either through program realignment or through people, will be a key to making it work.

POPULATIONS AT RISK

The long-term care population can be broken down roughly into three groups: those with chronic physical disease, the mentally retarded, and the chronic mentally ill. Many of the problems of these groups are not amenable to similar solutions. The intent here is to first isolate the various populations at risk, and to examine the size, characteristics, and service needs of each. Once we have identified these populations, we will be in a position to outline the common areas of need to which similar programmatic remedies might be applied.

Data in the areas of chronic impairments and unmet needs are fragmented and incomplete. What follows is an attempt to show something of the nature and magnitude of chronic impairments, within the limits of the data. Table 2.1 shows the numbers of institutionalized persons and estimates of noninstitutionalized persons at risk for long-term care.

The Aged

The aged as a group are particularly at risk for chronic conditions and resultant impairments, and resulting from the changing make-up of the aged population are likely to become even more so over the next decades. From 9 million in 1940 the aged grew to 20.2 million in 1970; projections show that by the year 2000 there will be nearly 30 million aged.[1]

The risk of chronic impairments grows among the over 75 age group and becomes especially high among the over 85 group—19 percent of those over 85 are in institutions. Elderly people who experience trauma such as widowhood and retirement also are highly at risk for institutionalization, a status that is rarely changed once it occurs in the elderly. Functional impairments, social isolation, poverty, and multiple conditions commonly occur among the aged, and all of them account for institutionalization, which among the elderly frequently occurs for social and economic reasons.

The Community

While the elderly in institutions have more chronic conditions than the elderly as a whole, there are many indications that there is an equivalent

TABLE 2.1

Populations in Institutions and at Risk in the Community

Nursing Homes (includes SNF and ICF)	1,200,000
Chronic Disease Hospitals	25,000
VA Hospitals (Psychotic—long stay)[a]	25,000
Psychiatric Hospitals	250,000
Institutions for the Mentally Retarded	200,000
Non-Institutional Population	
Mentally Retarded (substantially handicapped)	670,000
Aged Needing Care at Home	3,400,000
Severely Mentally Disordered	1,000,000
Developmentally Disabled[b]	
Cerebral Palsy	580,000
Epileptic	206,000
Other Neurological Disorders	600,000

[a]This represents a minimum rather than a total for all VA patients.

[b]Does not include other categories of severely physically impaired.

Sources: U.S. Department of Health. Education. and Welfare. *Health, United States, 1975*, p. 255; and Ethel Shanas. "Measuring the Home Health Needs of the Aged in Five Countries." *Journal of Gerontology* 26, no. 1 (1971), p. 38; Department of Health. Education. and Welfare. Public Health Service. "Changes in the Age, Sex and Diagnostic Composition of the Resident Population of State and County Mental Hospitals. U.S., 1964–1973." *Statistical Note 112*, DHEW Pubn. no. (ADM) 75-158 (1975). pp. 6–7; Murray Tucker. *Background and Analysis: Long-Term Care for the Mentally Retarded* (Washington. D.C.: The Urban Institute, 1975). p. 4; U.S. Department of Health. Education, and Welfare, National Institute of Mental Health. "The Severely Mentally Discordered." by Valerie J. Bradley for use of The White House Conference for Handicapped Individuals (1976). p. 15.

population in community settings. It may be that these people manage to keep out of institutions because of better family and financial resources, or that they simply cannot qualify for Medicaid reimbursement for nursing home care. It is difficult to describe services actually provided to the aged in the community, especially long-term care services. There are many specialized programs for the aged, but none meets a total need; for example, about 240,000 meals are served each day by the community nutrition program sponsored by the Administration on Aging, though the acknowledged need is much greater.

Limitations in physical performance and in independent living are most prevalent among the very aged population—those over age 75.[2] This group has been identified by many as the one most at risk for impairment and disease and most in need of services. They are called the "frail elderly," and have been singled out as the primary concern of the Federal Council on Aging. The frail elderly or aged patient who is over 75 has been defined as "partially ambulant or wheelchair bound, who needs super-vision in some activities such as bathing, assistance in other activities such as shopping or cleaning, and general surveillance such as in medical care."[3] There are an estimated 8 million people over age 75 in the United States, and a total of 22 million people over 65.[4]

The high incidence of limitations in mobility and independent living among the aged indicates a need for assistance of substantial proportions in the community. Since the functional limitations are frequently accom-panied by health problems, what is important is a combination of health and social, or personal care services. The service requirements among this population fluctuate, rather than remain static, so that in addition to an array of services, some continuing overview or monitoring is necessary to adapt services to changing status.

Estimates of aged persons in the community needing home care in-clude the bedfast and housebound, as well as those with less limiting conditions who have difficulty in getting about. Approximately 3.4 million aged persons, about 18 percent of the noninstitutionalized population, need some kind of home care and support on a continuing basis.[5] These services are not generally available, or if they are, the aged frequently cannot afford them. The necessary organizations to provide continuing assessment and monitoring are also lacking.

Institutions

Nursing home residents account for the bulk of the total institu-tionalized population—over 1 million out of a total of 1.6 million. Ninety percent of nursing home residents are over 65, 75 percent are over 75, and 38 percent are over 85. There are also approximately 70,000 aged patients in psychiatric hospitals.[6] Although about 1 million aged persons are in nursing homes at one time, about 20 percent of the aged—5 million—spend some time in a nursing home.

Institutional and community residents over age 65 who have any chronic impairments are likely to have multiple impairments, often a mix of physical and mental factors. The Public Health Service Report on *Health, United States, 1975* shows the major conditions of the institutionalized aged to be hardening of the arteries, "senility," stroke, and other mental disorders. The aged nursing home patient has an average of three chronic conditions.

Of those nursing home residents with heart trouble, cerebrovascular disease, arthritis or rheumatism, diabetes, senility, or arteriosclerosis, about 6.6 percent were confined totally to bed. The mobility level was consistently lowest for those with cerebrovascular disease (stroke). About 26 percent with these diseases were confined to bed part of the day, and to a wheelchair for the rest. About 12 percent used wheelchairs but required minimal help getting around, and another 17 percent were confined to the home but did not use a wheelchair. About 37 percent were able to leave the premises with or without assistance.[7]

Although an individual may have chronic conditions, the actual reason for nursing home placement is often the person's functional and self-care limitations, which may be residuals of the actual medical condition.

The availability of a spouse also appears to be a significant factor in institutionalization; among married couples in 1970 with living husband or wife aged 65 or over, fewer than 0.5 percent were institutionalized, whereas 7 percent of older nonmarried persons were institutionalized. Among the elderly, the group most at risk for institutionalization is the recently widowed (two years or less) female. Nearly two-thirds of patients in nursing and personal care homes in 1969 were widowed; 42 percent of the men were widowed, and 71 percent of the women.[8] These figures are important in that they illustrate the tendency toward institutionalization when the emotional and personal environment is disrupted, and not replaced by any community supports or other informal care.

Income is also a factor in the decision to enter a nursing home; resources are depleted, leaving the impaired person unable to purchase services outside the institution, and public assistance may be insufficient to sustain them at home. Two-thirds of skilled nursing and intermediate care facility patients are Medicaid recipients. They have either spent down to the poverty level, or they entered poor. One-quarter of the aged have incomes below the poverty level; 3 million Supplemental Security Income (SSI) recipients have incomes even lower, a fact which often makes Medicaid-supported nursing home care a desirable alternative to poverty and substandard housing.[9]

While social and economic factors influence the need for nursing home care, it is obvious that the population at risk also has substantial chronic disease and impairment. The population needs far more services than it receives in the nursing home, or than the facility is prepared to provide. Data from *Health, United States, 1975* on the nursing home population indicates that one-half of the patients have mental disorders, one-half cannot see to read, one-third cannot hear a telephone conversation, and one-third had no replacement for missing teeth. The patients had an average of three chronic diseases, and almost all had mobility limitations. We can compare these statistics on patient impairments with the statistics on the services the patients received: 10 percent received physical therapy, 6 percent received occupational therapy, 15 percent received recreational therapy, and 0.5 percent received speech therapy. Significantly, mental health care is not even listed as a service.

It is extremely difficult to compare services needed with services received, but it is apparent from the fragmentary evidence that maintenance, preventive, and therapeutic care are rarely provided in nursing homes. Physician visits to nursing home patients are usually infrequent. Of patients in a nursing home one year or more, 13 percent had not been seen by a physician in at least six months, and 9 percent had not been seen in more than a year. One-fourth of all nursing home patients had not been seen in the past three months (at the time of the survey, reported in *Health, United States, 1975*). In contrast, the aged population in the community saw a physician on the average of 6.5 times per year. It is strange that the nursing home population apparently receives less medical attention than the generally healthier aged population as a whole.

Intermediate care facilities (ICFs) contain populations ranging from those who could also qualify for skilled nursing care to those who need some kind of sheltered living environment. Indications are that most persons are in ICFs not for the purpose of receiving health care, but to receive domiciliary care.[10] Although most ICF residents do have one or more diagnosed chronic conditions, the average being three, not all are referred directly by physicians; many were self-referred and gave economic and social reasons for doing so. Their chronic conditions are generally stable, and they have generally high functional capacities, both mental and physical.

The Physically Disabled Adult

This group does not fit conveniently into any other category, for their total needs are quite different. These persons are generally quite severely disabled, and are dependent upon others for some or all activities of daily living. In spite of their impairments, however, they have the same expectations and desires as any other groups of their age.

Because of their continuous need for care, physically disabled persons are often placed in nursing homes for want of family or other resources. Aside from restricting personal freedom and liberty to move about and maintain relationships with peers, placement in a total institution usually precludes any possibility of employment or education. Even those living with and dependent on family support do not wish to continue this dependence.

The severely physically disabled are paraplegics, quadriplegics, some blind persons, and those with debilitating disease, such as multiple sclerosis, muscular dystrophy, and cerebral palsy. Onset of disability may occur at birth, or it may follow an illness such as polio, or a traumatic accident.

There are almost no data on the numbers of persons in this group, or on their residential and care status. We do know that the number is small, relative to the other major impaired populations. Their service needs are mostly of the personal care type: mobility, dressing, bathing, toileting. They are very dependent on others for physical activities, but not at all for supervision, nonroutine medical care, or income maintenance. They are employable at any job within their physical limits. In addition to personal care, or "attendant" needs, their major need may be for accessible housing, adapted to meet their needs for independent living.

Children and young adults with chronic conditions encounter unique problems. Many children who are severely crippled or have other chronic conditions stay for years in short-stay acute hospitals for lack of an alternative. Mentally retarded children, if their conditions are severe, disappear into large institutions for the duration of their lives. Physically handicapped or retarded adults are often placed in mental or other institutions upon the death of a parent or relative who had cared for them. These groups rarely have any independent income and are supported by parents or by the state. Young adults who are physically handicapped from such conditions as paralysis, cerebral palsy, or multiple sclerosis require at least some personal care, and some need income support. There are no special living arrangements for them except with families, and there is little income replacement available to them, except for SSI, for which they must first impoverish themselves. A few are able to qualify for disability insurance. The greatest economic impact of disability occurs among nonmarried, severely disabled persons; the majority of them fall below the poverty level. Thus, many young, physically handicapped persons have no choice but to live as public assistance recipients in nursing homes and other institutions where they can receive personal care services.

The Mentally Retarded and the Developmentally Disabled

Developmental disabilities are defined as attributable to mental retardation, cerebral palsy, epilepsy, or other related neurological conditions. They have been discovered and diagnosed before the individual reaches the age of 18 and constitute substantial handicaps. Mental retardation is defined on the basis of IQ, as well as adaptive behavior. The estimated number of mentally retarded persons of all ages in the United States is 6 million, of whom an estimated 670,000 are severely handicapped. Among the rest of the developmentally disabled population, there are an estimated 580,000 cerebral palsied, 206,000 epileptics, and 600,000 with other neurological disorders including muscular dystrophy and speech and hearing disorders.

In terms of functional impairments, the profoundly retarded are almost totally impaired. They are unable to move about or care for themselves, need total care, and are not easily able to reside in a family setting unless the family makes inordinate sacrifices. Beyond this group, the variables are numerous: the severely or moderately retarded person might have varying degrees of ability to manage some personal care chores under supervision. The mildly retarded, depending on emotional and behavioral stability, do not usually live in institutions, are often able to care for themselves, and many hold jobs. They might be able to live in a sheltered environment or alone.

Approximately 238,000 mentally retarded. persons reside in institutions; of these, 181,000 or 75 percent were in public institutions; 28,000 or 12 percent in private institutions, and 30,000 or 13 percent were in state mental hospitals. [11] The great majority of the institutionalized retarded are the more severely or profoundly retarded; studies have shown that most of this population is below the mildly retarded level or below an IQ of 55. The noninstitutionalized population is weighted toward the more mildly and moderately impaired. [12]

Increased emphasis on community residential settings for the retarded means that those remaining in institutions will be mostly the severely and profoundly retarded. They need a high degree of custodial care, as well as medical and rehabilitative services, and there is little turnover for this group. Discharge is usually by death, and the median length of stay by an adult aged 19–64 in an institution for the mentally retarded is over 16 years.

There has been increasing emphasis on "deinstitutionalization" or discharging the mentally retarded to families, foster homes, halfway houses, or other community settings. There is a lack of such community and supportive services for those who cannot be fully independent. Some 250,000 mentally retarded noninstitutionalized individuals received some services (other than education) in 1971, out of a total substantially handicapped population of about 700,000 and a total retarded population of 6 million. Educational programs have been excluded from this study. Day services are available for some mentally retarded; about 2,000 facilities provide day care. Of these, 484 include sheltered workshops, 1,341 include personal care services, 1,406 provide training, 745 provide education, 104 provide diagnosis and evaluation, and 193 provide treatment. About 92,000 noninstitutionalized mentally retarded were served by these centers in 1970. [13] Another 71,000 were served in mental retardation clinics (evaluation and treatment), 37,000 in outpatient psychiatric clinics, and 15,000 in community mental health centers. Thirty-one thousand were served in vocational rehabilitation programs. Many of these programs are unevenly distributed geographically, and they do not all provide comprehensive services.

The Mentally Ill

While there are many persons limited in their emotional performance who never receive active treatment for their problems, there is a subgroup of the mentally ill population who is both severely and chronically mentally disordered, and who will be in and out of institutions much of their lives. These people are substantially limited in the activities they can undertake; they are dependent, frequently unemployable, and have low incomes. They need treatment, care and protective services over a long period of time. Their conditions may be chronic, or they may be reversible; in either case they are long term. Their difficulty in dealing with the world and their problems in holding jobs make them additionally dependent upon others; long periods of institutionalization exacerbate this. The usual diagnoses for the long-term mental patient are psychoses, schizophrenia, and chronic or organic irreversible brain syndromes.

While there are no specific data to give an exact count of the number of seriously mentally disturbed persons in the country, available research estimates indicate a population of between 1 million and 1.5 million persons.[14]

The incidence of mental illness increases with age, with persons over age 75 most often reporting severe emotional limitations.[15] Estimates of mental impairment among the aged run as high as 15 to 20 percent, at least in the urban aged, and this impairment is often chronic in nature.[16]

Most of the data currently collected describes institutional populations and the use of certain community mental health resources rather than the populations using them. Therefore, the following is more a description of services than of populations.

Inpatient Care

There are 570 psychiatric hospitals in the United States: 354 state and local, 31 Veterans Administration, 95 proprietary, and 90 private nonprofit. The number of beds has remained relatively stable for the last three categories: about 13,117 in 1974.[17] The state hospitals accounted for 280,277 inpatient beds in 1974, down 22 percent from 1972. This is part of the continuing deinstitutionalization being carried on by the states; in spite of these efforts, state hospitals still account for the bulk of the total 393,394 beds. Although the number of beds available is close to 400,000, the actual patient census in 1973 was actually around 250,000, reflecting the surplus of beds as a result of deinstitutionalization efforts.

The average size of the public psychiatric hospital is about 2,000 patients, similar to institutions for the mentally retarded. The two groups share problems in addition to size, such as inadequate budgets, lack of staff and treatment, and outdated facilities. The most frequent diagnoses of resident inpatients are schizophrenia (the vast majority), mental retardation, and organic brain syndrome (usually associated with cerebral arteriosclerosis).[18] Not surprisingly, organic brain syndrome is usually associated with the aged, while schizophrenia is more evenly spread across age groups. Although the age of the institutionalized population has shifted somewhat toward the younger side because of transfer of many aged patients to nursing homes and other settings, the aged still account for a substantial portion—28 percent—of this population.

Psychiatric hospitals, particularly public ones, are essentially long-stay facilities for many patients. While most inpatient "episodes" are relatively brief, there occurs what looks like a sedimentation effect. Out of each group of admissions, some will settle down to stay a long time. Surveys done by Arthur Bolton Associates in Virginia, Pennsylvania, and New Jersey showed the following averages: 22.8 percent of the state hospital residents had been there for 1 to 5 years; 12.8 percent for 5 to 10 years, and 42 percent for over 10 years.[19]

While many patients, even long-stay ones, have been released, the residue consists of many who have been there such a long time that they have nowhere else to go. Of those who are released, chances of return are high. In addition to the residents of psychiatric institutions, over half of all nursing home residents are reported to have some kind of mental or emotional disorder. While not all of these disorders are severe, they are rarely treated in nursing homes and, thus, cannot be expected to improve.

Outpatient Services

Many inpatient psychiatric facilities currently provide outpatient services, usually to those who have been released from inpatient status. The future trend will likely be toward more outpatient care as institutions attempt to provide better services to those patients released in the cause of deinstitutionalization who now receive little support. In 1971, outpatient units were maintained in 312 hospitals, and 253 had partial hospitalization programs where an individual could go to the hospital either on a day or night basis while living or working in the community. Home care programs existed in 33 institutions in 1971, and there were over 100 psychiatric foster care programs maintained by hospitals.

' Halfway houses for the ex-mental patient have become popular in concept, if not in actual application; there were 209 psychiatric halfway houses in 1973, and 6,000 persons resided in them.[20] The median stay in these facilities is 11 months; during this time work and community life adjustments can be made and therapy and counseling received. In addition to halfway houses, there are various protective living settings, which are not widely available, and are of mixed value. These include supervised apartments, boarding homes, and group homes.

Psychiatric outpatient facilities are available in some hospitals, and community mental health centers (CMHC) provide some services, although there are only 500 CHMCs out of an originally projected total of 2,000 or more. Not only are they unavailable to much of the population, but CHMCs and other outpatient facilities have often failed to treat chronic and ex-mental patients.

Little information on services offered in the community is available, except that they are scattered and inadequate. There are many ideas about services *needed*. A range of community-based residential services, and rehabilitative services of both psychic and vocational natures, are cited.[21] Other services needs include social support and activities, case management, service continuity, assistance to families in caring for the mentally disordered, coping skills, normalization, and advocacy.[22]

A COORDINATED SYSTEM OF LONG TERM CARE

Introduction

Having arrived at an understanding of the magnitude of the long-term care problem we can proceed to consider the components of an effective system of care. While our survey of the populations at risk may suggest that the groups that fall into the long-term care category are very diverse, they, in fact, share a need for certain kinds and combinations of service.

Briefly, all of the population groups contain segments needing institutional care, sheltered living arrangements in the community, or home care. A good selection of health, social, and income services is needed in addition to the variety of living settings. Although the emphasis and intensity of the services might vary among the groups, the nature of many of the services and settings would not. Thus, there is reason to believe that some of the needs of differing populations could be met through the same mechanisms and by the same service providers.

Patterns of Management and Treatment

Evidence of common areas of need among the various populations at risk is furnished by the treatment and management patterns for chronic conditions. These patterns can be clearly distinguished from the treatment patterns for acute illness and serve to point up the existence of certain service needs consistent for a wide variety of chronic conditions. An acute illness occurs suddenly and is usually resolved in a short period of time through medication, surgery, or the simple course of the illness. Chronic conditions, on the other hand, are often gradual in onset, except when caused by trauma or congenital factors, and until an acute flare-up occurs, can often be barely perceptible. They are difficult, frequently impossible, to treat, and they are of lifelong duration. Medical intervention is limited to maintaining the status quo or effecting some functional improvements. Chronic conditions may also be characterized by recurring acute episodes that are treated in the same manner as any other acute condition.

The chronic condition is also characterized by different patterns of health care utilization—higher incidence of long-term institutional use and more hospitalizations. The length of stay in institutions for chronic physical or mental conditions is also much greater.

An individual with one chronic condition is often saddled with multiple ailments. This can be a function of older age, for the elderly, as we have seen, are very much at risk for multiple chronic conditions. One condition can often contribute to the development of another; for example, chronic kidney disease may help cause heart problems. Thus, the treatment difficulties presented by a chronically ill patient are different from and more complex over a long period of time than an acute illness, which may require high technical skills for a brief period.

The cost of long-term care is usually higher than acute care, both because of the variety of services required and their duration. Often the chronically ill individual with more than one condition, or with complex needs, must see numerous specialists and obtain a variety of services. The cost to the individual is much greater, for much of this is not covered by an insurance program. Medicare, for example, is an acute care benefit and provides little relief from the burdens of chronic illness. The out-of-pocket medical care cost to the aged in 1974 averaged $1,200; in addition, cost to both the individual and society is reflected in the partial or total loss of ability to earn money. The acute illness, on the other hand, may result in temporary loss of ability to work, but income is frequently replaced by workers' compensation and other short-term, stop-gap programs.

Finally, because of its complex medical, economic, and social effects, chronic disease requires substantial management and coordination efforts. Periodic screening for other conditions is needed, and the use of a variety of specialized services and drugs must be monitored. These services are rarely coordinated among practitioners, partly due to the lack of administrative units within which this can occur, the distaste of physicians and other health professionals for management, the heavy demands on these providers' time, and the fragmentation of care brought about by the increase in specialization. Health care is not routinely coordinated with income or social service programs. Thus, the chronically ill person with long-term health care needs is typically cared for in an acute care environment which is fragmented, medically oriented, and specialized. It is a sickness-oriented system, not a health-oriented one that would consider the total client.

A Framework for a System of Long-Term Care

We have seen that chronic conditions of various kinds are alike to the extent that they are difficult to treat, are often accompanied by other ailments, and may have complex economic and social ramifications for the individual. An effective system of long-term care must take into account the multiple needs of this population and provide a comprehensive range of services and supports to meet those needs.

Objectives of Care

We can define an overall goal for long-term care as the promotion of the greatest possible level of physical, social, and psychological functioning in the chronically ill and impaired population. This entails helping the individual to maintain the highest capacity for independence, whether in the community or in an institution, and helping the individual to remain in the most normal environment for his or her capacities. These objectives can be achieved by preventing loss of functional abilities, minimizing the effect of the loss of those abilities when it occurs, and rehabilitating to the maximum capacity level.

What is needed to do these things is a package of services and supports designed to provide diagnostic, therapeutic, rehabilitative, maintenance, and monitoring services.

Services Needed

Common service needs of disabled and chronically ill populations are broken down in this way.

1. *Health services*: physician, nursing, screening, outpatient, therapeutic, and nutrition services.

2. *Personal care services*: home health aide, homemaker, attendant, assistance with daily living activities such as walking, shopping, dressing, and bathing.

3. *Support services*: transportation, meals, social integration, psychological support and therapy, vocational rehabilitation, and social services.

4. *Housing of various types*: protective living arrangements, congregate housing, institutional care.

5. *Services which cover a variety of need categories*: day hospital, adult day services, respite care (availability of services to give respite to family or attendant).

6. *Money to purchase needed food, shelter, and services.*

The effective delivery of the services described must also be assured. The chronically ill or impaired individual must have access to the right services when needed, and accessibility is a product of many factors: money, transportation, mobility, information, timing, availability, and competence in the delivery system.

Service Coordination

Not only is there a need for a range of effectively delivered services, but there is a need to develop a *system* of care that would provide continuous and well-coordinated services to the long-term care population. The fragmented nature of programs and funding makes coordination the major requirement of human services. It would be impossible, of course, to place all of the services required by the long-term care population under a single administrative roof; there are simply too many of them, and they are too diverse. The need, however, is to make the providers flexible enough at the top level to be amenable to coordination and the meeting of human needs at the service level.

The Need for Coordination and Assessment

Current programs attempt to deal with appropriateness, efficiency, and proper use of institutional care through mechanisms that usually function after decisions have already been made about the type of service and setting to be delivered. The decision is a reimbursement one, and the enforcement of the above criteria implies a rational medical decision. Such mechanisms hardly even exist for community services. Such indirect attempts at assessment as utilization review, preadmission authorization, and claims review are really attempts to control utilization without making an assessment of client needs. Decisions about these things are often impossible to correct after the fact. Incomplete information about the client often results in the wrong choice of program, services, reimbursement, and setting. In a large proportion of cases, community services and supports are not considered; hospital discharge planners and physicians often favor institutional placements instead.

Most proposals for reform in long-term care have suggested a service coordination vehicle combined with an assessment mechanism to eliminate these problems, on the assumption that any adequate assessment of care and placement needs must occur before fiscal decisions are made. It is believed that in the past, financing decisions have preceded and governed these other decisions.

Past Experience

Many social service professionals and researchers—as well as government policymakers—view service integration as the key to coordination. Integration is the building of systems of service, either through voluntary cooperation or the use of specific power to promote cooperation.[23] The use of contracting authority, case managers, and pooled funding have also been tried with some success, though without conclusive results.

The effects of these attempts to rationalize services upon the populations to be served have not been thoroughly evaluated. No specific formulas for coordination or integration have been judged successful and generally replicable, although some interesting prospects have been raised, and some are beginning to be tested. The Services Integration for Deinstitutionalization (SID) project conducted in Virginia, for example, found that coordination among state level agencies only functioned when formalized by explicit interagency contracts and that centralized authority was essential to the effort's success.[24]

Much of the literature dealing with service coordination limits discussion to "social services" rather than health services or health and social services. Yet the provision of health care is frequently essential to the success of social service delivery and vice versa; the coordination of health with social—and economic—services is as important as coordination among an array of social services.

Purpose and Functions

The purpose of coordination and assessment is to increase the effectiveness and efficiency of categorical and specialized programs and funding sources and to reduce the human and fiscal costs of inappropriate treatment and placement. Services and settings would be used in accordance with the individual's situation and requirements—in the right place, at the right time. Existing resources would be used wherever possible to avoid duplication, and fragmentation of services could be reduced.

An assessment-coordination system would perform a number of functions, beginning with *evaluation and diagnosis*. The evaluation would include an assessment of client status, service needs, eligibility status, and coverage. One individual might administer the initial screening, making use of a reliable assessment tool. A team of professionals would then evaluate the results of the screening and make recommendations. The next step, *prescription*, would take into account the primary care physician evaluation and would involve recommendations to the client concerning a course of action and a service or package of services. The client would be advised of such matters as service setting, program eligiblity requirements, and out-of-pocket costs. The coordination-assessment service would then make *referrals* and, if necessary, make contact with and brief service providers. *Follow-up* would also be the responsibility of the service; the service would act as an agent for the client in seeing that prescribed services were actually received. In addition, periodic reassessments of client status and progress would be carried out as part of the follow-up. The health of the client and other factors would be subject to *continuous monitoring*, so that changes which might indicate different service requirements could be detected.

One additional function of the assessment coordination system would be *representation and mediation*. The system would have the responsibility of following up complaints and advising providers when reassessments indicate that insufficient, inappropriate, or poor quality services are being rendered. Here the system could function as an ombudsman for the client.

Methods of Coordination

It is difficult to specify an overall model for community coordination on a nationwide basis because much depends on local characteristics and resources. In what follows, we simply set forth several alternative models for a community assessment and coordination system.

Independent Community Agency. This model would be a community-based service independent of public and private service agencies and providers and composed of a multidisciplinary team of professional and technical personnel.

The service could be financed in a number of ways: (a) through payment by federally assisted programs that provide third party payments for related services, supplemented by fees from clients able to pay. Capitation payments could be the method of reimbursement, based on the potential population at risk in the community; (b) special funding from local revenues, state contributions, and special federal funding. This could be done on a block grant or capitation basis; or (c) initial assessment could be reimbursed by health insurance programs, either national or other, as diagnostic services.

The independent model would meet certain staffing and competence criteria in order to receive any public funds and would accept clients who are self-referred or referred by providers and other agencies. The recommendations of the service would not be binding on the client.

The service would maintain a relationship with the local health systems agency, making recommendations about needed resources and services, based on its assessment and referral experience.

Agency Coalitions. Under this model, there would be a community-based council composed of a coalition of existing public, private, and voluntary service agencies. This model, instead of being independent, would depend on member agencies for support and staff. Funding would come from general revenues and third party program payments. The coalitions would have to be mandated by federal or state law and given sufficient powers and funding to make them work.

In addition to the functions described for the independent agency, this one would also be authorized and responsible for determining its clients' eligibility for public programs and services. Thus, service availability would be assured, and referrals would constitute authorization for services. Although the community council would not have direct responsibility for utilization review or health planning, representatives of review and planning functions should be members of the coalition, and coalition members should participate in planning and review functions.

The coalition, instead of being completely autonomous, might have to be given some authority and impetus, either by direction from a statewide body, or by virtue of the authority to make its decisions binding, subject only to client wishes.

Needless to say, the possibility of breakdowns is a major problem with coalitions, but it is possible that this could be overcome in some localities, particularly if contracts are used.

Single Public Agency. A single existing agency, state or local, could be designated as the service coordinator-client evaluator and perform the same functions as the independent agency. The agency, such as the health department, social services, or other agency, would be given responsibility and funding by the local government to make its referrals binding on other service providers (if such referrals are desired by the client) and on the staff of its own agency. The agency authorized to act in this capacity would have to create a separate arm to perform the function.

The reluctance of the other agencies and providers to accept the authority of this service could be a major problem, as could the development of multidisciplinary work in a single agency setting.

Assessment and Planning. This model could be either an independent local agency or a coalition, but would have the added authority to identify, develop, and allocate services and resources. This would include resource planning authority in conjunction with, but not dependent upon, the health systems agencies, for monitoring quality and establishing criteria for local services. It could also determine individual eligibility.

There are problems as well as advantages in lodging too many functions in one place; one agency could become too controlling, and begin to restrict or pervert the use of services.

Contracting Arrangements. Any of the above agencies could, in lieu of the authority to make their decisions binding on other agencies, work with the client to make binding contracts with other agencies for the provision of services. The contracts would be worked out in a way that is satisfactory to both the client and provider.

COMMUNITY SERVICES AND INSTITUTIONAL PLACEMENT

The development of a system of long-term care will call for some reassessment of the roles of the community and the institution in providing services to the chronically ill and impaired population. In this section, we examine the issue of appropriate placement and trace some of the relevant developments in institutional and community care. While the current demand for "alternatives" to the institution may make the two types of settings appear to be mutually exclusive, efforts to single out one form of care that could supplant the institution would only be misspent. The real objective for policymakers should be to build a complex of services combining the resources of the institution with those of the community. An exchange or integration of services would have a twofold advantage: it would facilitate the selection of a range of services best suited to the needs of the individual, and it would help to eliminate the costly duplication and fragmentation of services which characterize the long-term care system at present.

Appropriate Setting for Care

Decisions about whether a person should be cared for in an institution, at home, or in some community setting, can be made on the basis of the variety and intensity of services needed, as well as on the basis of cost. If the person needs constant supervision and surveillance, an institutional setting may be required; if the patient needs sporadic health services, nonprofessional therapy, meals, or some personal care assistance, the home may be a more desirable and efficient care setting.*

---

*It should be noted that this discussion assumes equal availability and funding for various settings; this is a desired model, not a program-oriented one.

The first site considered should be the individual's home setting. If there are family supports available, some nonskilled services could be provided by the family. Or the person may live in housing that has some personal care services available. Other services requiring professional application or supervision could be brought to the individual or the individual to them, that is, home health care, day care, rehabilitation, outpatient care, and so on. Where family or other support is not available, some personal assistance services may need to be added on an intermittent basis (homemaker, meals, shopping, bathing, ambulation).

Persons in community living arrangements whose needs become continuous and intensive, and whose needs must be met by outside agencies, might be more efficiently cared for in an institutional setting—unless such needs are considered to be relatively short-term. The category of institution would depend on the type and mix of services needed.

In making the decision to place someone in an institution many factors need to be considered. For policymakers and program operators, the important criterion will be how much it costs their program or how much it will cost the public. This question is not answerable with solid data yet. Indications, based on demonstrations and research, are that home health services—even intensive ones—on an intermittent or sporadic basis—are less costly than their institutional counterparts.

Issues of "Appropriate Placement"

A partial answer to the question of the appropriate care setting can be found in the desires of the patients themselves, regardless of regulatory considerations. A study of nursing home patients in Hillsborough County, Florida, revealed that 85 percent of the patients questioned said they would rather remain in their homes.[25] This response is hardly surprising in view of the current public image of nursing homes as corrupt, dirty, uncaring, and in view of the fact that the nursing home is a total institution in the sense that a prison is—personal freedoms are severely restricted and old habits must be given up.

Other studies have postulated that a significant number of long-term care facility patients are inappropriately placed based on their care needs. Depending on criteria for service needs used, figures range from 15 to 80 percent for inappropriate nursing home placement. Since none of the available studies used the same measurements and criteria, it is not possible to reach any definite conclusions about the magnitude of the problem.[26] Based on actual surveys indicating levels of care received by patients, it may be reasonable to place the figure at about 30 percent, since no systematic evaluation has ever been done.[27]

The problems of appropriate placement have been compounded by federal funding requirements, mainly those of Medicaid. Patients were frequently—and still are—placed in nursing homes even though they did not actually need that level of care in order to obtain Medicaid reimbursement which was not available elsewhere. From 1965 to 1971, Medicaid reimbursed states on a matching basis for care in skilled nursing facilities (then called skilled nursing homes); lower levels such as boarding or personal care homes were not reimbursed by Medicaid. Intermediate care facilities (ICFs) were not eligible for vendor payments, but relied on payment out of the resident's cash grant under the public assistance programs. The tendency in the states was to place patients in skilled nursing facilities (SNFs) to obtain federal matching; there was no utilization review to control this practice at the time, and there were few choices for the individual. In 1971, in order to create a lower level and lower cost alternative to the SNF, Congress acted to remove the ICF from the welfare program and place it in Medicaid as part of a continuum of care. It was anticipated that many patients would be reclassified to this lower level of care.

The ICF program also includes health-related parts of public institutions for the mentally retarded. Currently, there are no systematic data on these facilities, though there are indications of placement problems here as well—in addition to the whole deinstitutionalization question. This is the first time federal matching funds have been available to these institutions, and it is possible that policies may be stretched to include residents whether or not they are in need of or receiving an active health care program. Advocacy groups have expressed their concern that the regulations establish false levels of care by encouraging providers to classify residents who are only in need of sheltered living and habilitation as recipients of health care.

The problem of inappropriate placement has not been solved by the ICF program; people still end up in institutions because they need assistance with activities of daily living or a place to live and there is nothing for them in the community. Placement in a long-term care institution appears to depend a great deal on available funding sources, or on a physician's or hospital's recommendation; they will commonly recommend a nursing home because it is simplest for them to arrange, and they are often unaware of other alternatives.[28] Medical conditions, functional limitations, and the availability of family or other help also enter into decisions, though these aspects often become secondary to current funding policies on the part of the states. At least one state has reportedly reduced to almost zero its approval of Medicaid reimbursement for patients in skilled nursing facilities, and other states have imposed similar restrictions, including reduced reimbursement rates, in efforts to control costs.[29]

Unfortunately, the squeeze can come from both ends; most states provide minimal reimbursement for Medicaid home health services; California, for example, has reduced this program to almost nothing. The individual is thus forced to rely on cash programs or to go to an institutional form of care.

Developments in Community Care

The development of a system of long-term care and the reduction of institutional use to those who can be served in no other way have been hindered by the lack of additional resources for providing services in the communities. These factors, coupled with poor conditions in many institutions, produced a desire to find "alternatives." The word became the symbol of an undefined need for new ways of providing services. While the use of such a general word may suggest an inability to articulate the specifics of different policy, the need to control costs of institutional care and to find a more desirable and humane way of caring for the aged and impaired population is evident. There has been a shift in emphasis from the desire to find a place for people who need help to the desire to find the right place and the right help.

It seems apparent that no single "alternative" provides the answer. In terms of savings, while some or all of them may be less costly than institutional care, the initial development of the resources will undoubtedly require substantial investment. In addition, it is important to consider that the impact of a system of community services on the utilization of nursing home care will not be measurable for a few years; it will not be possible to remove most patients from nursing homes, but we can slow the rate of admissions.

The use of the term, "alternatives to institutional care," is said by Brahna Trager to be: ". . . an attempt to express the search for services which make the combination—personal choice-appropriateness-economy—possible, and this does not exclude the use of the long- or short-term institution; it represents an *addition* of care components that allows for great dilution in some approaches and greater concentration in others—*with appropriateness as the decisive factor.*"[30] It is clear that instead of seeking "alternatives" we really need to develop a system of comprehensive services that are widely available in the community as well as in institutional settings.

Home Health Care

A comprehensive way to define home health care is to say that it is an array of services that may be brought into the home singly or in combination in order to achieve and sustain the optimum state of health, activity, and independence for individuals of all ages who require such services because of acute illness, exacerbations of chronic illness, or long-term permanent limitations due to chronic illness and disability.[31]

Much of the disagreement about home health care centers around the question of whether it should be a medical service or a social service. Medical services were viewed as skilled nursing services, physical therapy, and medical equipment. The "social" aspect of care was thought to be the personal care and homemaker-types of service; one was proper for health insurance and programs, the other was not. There is a growing realization, however, that the two must combine to form a health service; the medical service alone cannot keep a chairbound person independent; the social service cannot mitigate a medical condition.

Related to the social versus medical care debate is the level of care debate. There are many levels of home care, reflecting variations in the frequency and numbers of different services provided. For example, intensive services might include a complex of services: physician visits, daily nursing visits, physical therapy, equipment, and homemaker-home health aide services. The lower levels would differ only in that perhaps fewer services would be provided, and possibly, though not necessarily, less often.

Various types of agencies currently provide home care: hospital-based home health agencies, visiting nurse associations, public health departments, and homemaker-home health aide services. The clientele includes children and new mothers, the impaired aged, and the physically disabled.

The case of a 69-year-old woman who was paralyzed in her right side by a stroke provides an example of the type of client who can benefit from the home health care programs. The woman was bedridden, incontinent, and unable to do anything for herself. Her husband was considerably older than she, and both had come to the United States within the past two years; he was unaccustomed to doing any household work or shopping. Over the next few years a home health agency provided physical therapy, assistance, and retraining in self-care and activities of daily living, occupational therapy, nutrition and meal planning, and homemaker-home health aide services. Specific service areas included toilet training, ambulation, motivation, physical therapy for arm and leg mobility, fitting for leg brace, and assistance in finding adequate housing. The homemaker-aide provided almost daily exercises, ambulation, and therapy.

From her prior state of complete helplessness and despair, the woman learned to walk, use stairs, feed herself, do some cooking and light chores, and do needlework with her uninvolved hand. She was again fully continent. The husband had been able to cope with the agency's assistance and had learned to shop and cook. The couple was in and out of home care for several years, and currently receives very little assistance. Without the assistance they received, this couple clearly would not have been able to live in the community.

Day Services and Treatment

There are many variations on the theme of providing day services out of the home in order to avoid dependence and the need for placement in a total institution. Whatever the variation, the concept has long been established and used in Great Britain. The earliest arrival here was the day hospital—or night hospital—for the mentally ill. The patient would be allowed to live in and work outside, or live at home and receive treatment in the hospital.

Day care services for other adult populations have more recently gained popularity here. At the most highly specialized end of the spectrum is the day hospital, for people who need medical and rehabilitative services on an intensive basis, but who do not need round-the-clock care and supervision. Adult day health centers, or day treatment centers, provide less intensive services than day hospitals, but still concentrate on providing therapeutic and health-oriented services to the aged or impaired adult. Typically, these centers provide preliminary assessments, health care, personal care, nutrition, and social services.

Since "day care" implies custodial services only, there is a need to differentiate among those which provide custodial or recreational services only and those whose main purpose is to provide medical and health services. However, even day "social" centers are not really custodial in the sense of baby-sitting, or board and care homes; they do usually provide active services, such as occupational therapy, socialization, and nutrition. This need to differentiate among types is felt most acutely by those concerned with publicly financed programs. Many of these people feel that social care should not be financed through health programs.

Day care is seen by many as a less expensive alternative to the total institution; however, we must be certain that services of like type are compared. For example, it would be inappropriate to compare costs of day hospital services to care in an intermediate care facility. It is also clear that day hospitals and day health centers cannot alone provide alternatives to institutional care for most people. If a person is seriously impaired, the practicality of remaining at home depends on the availability of other supports, such as family, home health, or homemaker services.

Community Living and Support Services

As a result of desires for greater availability of and access to community care, a variety of living arrangements and supportive services have emerged. Most of these are available only on a very small scale at the present time. For the individual who is not in need of institutional care, but for various reasons cannot live alone, protective or sheltered living can be a solution. It represents a middle ground between the community (of which it should be an integral part) and the institution. Many persons currently living in institutions could appropriately be placed in this environment. Domiciliary care homes, halfway houses, group homes for a variety of populations, adult foster homes, and some board and care homes are included in this category. Many homes for the aged provide room, board, and assistance or the assurance of help should it be needed. The severely physically handicapped often find this halfway step between nursing homes or other institutions and independent community life useful.

Adequate housing in general is essential to maintaining the independence of the impaired population. Safe, comfortable housing, and housing adapted to the special needs of some impaired persons, along with usable transportation, must be included in the spectrum of elements in independent living and maintenance of health.

The halfway house, or group home, serves as a permanent or transitional residence for ex-mental patients and other mentally disabled. Some of these homes provide an array of rehabilitation and social services, while others provide housekeeping and some supervision, or personal care services.

Adult foster homes are intended to provide family-type supports for aged persons unable to live alone, or for ex-mental patients. Boarding homes are also the frequent repository for "deinstitutionalized" patients. They provide shelter and meals but they do not offer personal care services. The fact that these facilities have changed little is probably due to the nature of the clientele; it has no funds to pay for services, and little voice to demand them. While the halfway/group home becomes more popular and better staffed, the boarding home remains shabby and unnoticed, the last home of many old people, and for the mentally ill a brief stay before inability to cope forces a return to the institution.

Another interesting trend in the development of protective living arrangements has emerged as a result of the severely physically disabled population's desire for self-determination and independence. Group homes, apartments modified to meet the needs of the disabled, and similar arangements have begun to emerge, bringing this group of young and middle-aged adults out of nursing homes or away from their parents to independent settings with the care and attendance needed. The development of these arrangements has been sporadic, though persistent; there are no specific funding arrangements for them, and some ingenuity is usually needed to find capital for operating expenses. Of course, much of this population is employed so there are funds available to lessen the reliance on public funds.

In addition to the supervised living arrangements, some of the facilities provide job training and health services. The group homes provide attendant services to those who need them, or they operate referral services. Group homes can consist of a complex of mutually managed apartments or a single shared residence. Services are made available as needed, and management is often shared by the residents themselves.

Developments in Institutional Services

There has been growing pressure for change in the long-term care field from the federal, state, and local levels, and from consumers and advocate groups. Finding alternatives to institutions has been a major concern, not only because of financing crises, but because long-term care institutions have developed in ways that are not considered desirable. Although nursing homes, psychiatric hospitals, and mental retardation institutions developed differently, all are now objects of concern about inappropriate placement, normalization (deinstitutionalization), and community service systems. One other fact seems to unite all of the facilities: they have developed, and continue, largely outside of the mainstream of health care delivery systems.

Nursing Homes:

This is a generic term for a broad group of facilities—including the skilled nursing facility, the intermediate care facility, the personal care home, and the domiciliary care facility—which provide care ranging from quasi-hospital to little more than room and board with some personal care. Regardless of the name or type of care, the nursing home developed from the social welfare residences and alms houses for the poor and incompetent. The concept was brought to this country from England with the settlers, who had grown up under the Elizabethan poor laws, and similar laws were passed establishing some public support for the residents of the homes.[32]

The "poor houses" and welfare homes were gradually forced into the provision of some health-related care and did so in spite of the fact that they remained outside the mainstream of health care, having no contact with hospitals and little with physicians.[33] Hospitals began to use them to relieve themselves of their chronically ill patients, thus placing a further health care burden on social care institutions. Public assistance programs indirectly supported them through cash payments to clients who in turn purchased care here.

Unlike the rest of the health care system, nursing home care has been characterized by an almost total lack of governmental interference. Recently this has been changed somewhat as a result of attention to physical and safety standards. The nursing home industry has always been mostly proprietary, though state and local governments and voluntary agencies also operated some; proprietary involvement has ballooned since the inception of Medicare and Medicaid, which provide a stable funding source. These same programs also forced existing facilities into an increasingly health-oriented role, so although the nursing homes frequently benefited from the business and profits they received, they had to struggle to provide services for which they were not equipped and for which they did not wish to divert profits. The result was a litany of scandals: fires, malnutrition, kickbacks, drug abuse, lack of medical care, and fraud.[34] It was not until 1969 that Medicaid was required to set standards of care in the 7,500 facilities in the program, and not until the 1970s did Medicare and Medicaid act to try to enforce standards. Later, recognition was given to the fact that facility and regulatory needs had been placed above the patients', and that issues of types and quality of care had to be resolved too.*

Institutions for Mental Illness and Mental Retardation:

Contrary to the nursing home, which is generally small (under 100 beds) and privately owned, these facilities have developed as very large, generally state-run institutions. These specialty institutions, however, also developed largely to solve social rather than health problems and to separate certain individuals from their normal environments. The states have built these facilities as "total" institutions: the resident is not free to mingle in the community. There was, at least in the psychiatric hospitals, some treatment, though rarely for the chronically ill "back ward" patients. The staffs of these facilities and large institutions for the retarded were frequently ill-trained, and included foreign-born and foreign-educated medical personnel who had difficulty communicating with residents. The facilities were subject to state budget constraints and services, and improvements here were usually the first to be cut. During the 1950s the use of chemotherapy resulted in a reduction of the institutionalized mentally ill population; in the 1960s scandals of poor quality institutional care and the growing belief that people were better treated in smaller facilities resulted in the movement to deinstitutionalize the retarded and mentally ill. Smaller

---

*Government efforts to regulate the nursing home industry are treated more fully in Hirsch Ruchlin's chapter, "An Analysis of Regulatory Issues and Options in Long-Term Care," Chapter 4 in this volume.

facilities for the mentally ill were built in some states, more services were brought in, and more people were released into "the community," though frequently without support services or follow-up.

The federal court system entered the area of institutional and community care in 1972 with the *Wyatt* vs. *Stickney* decision, which required the State of Alabama to improve its mental instititutions, release those residents who did not need to be confined, and to provide them with community services.

Reversing Trends

In the last several years concern about the quality of treatment and life in long-term care institutions has been increasing. Ways are being sought to curb the explosive growth of nursing home costs and facilities, and to find less restrictive ways of caring for the mentally ill, retarded, aged, and impaired. The primary question has become what is the right setting for providing care to an individual.

The "deinstitutionalization" movement began in the mental health field in the 1960s with the development of professionals' belief that the large mental hospital was not the most appropriate place of care for many of the patients housed there. In some areas the large state hospitals began to reorganize into smaller units; in some others, community clinics and halfway houses were developed.

Numerous studies have indicated that many patients could be appropriately placed in settings other than a state hospital. Two studies of patients in Texas mental institutions, one in 1966, the second in 1974, estimated that number to be about 50–65 percent of the resident population.[35] Other studies have estimated inappropriate placement of the aged in mental institutions to be even higher—well over 80 percent.[36] The 1974 Texas study indicated that 38 percent of the residents could be released, the majority of these (22 percent) to live in halfway houses or foster care homes. Another 26 percent were recommended for transfer to other facilities, primarily nursing homes. Over half (56 percent) of those recommended for transfer were over 60 years old, and 24 percent between 50 and 60. Most were long-term patients; one-half had been hospitalized for more than five years, and 30 percent for one to five years.[37]

These figures illustrate an important issue which affects nursing homes to a large degree. The enactment of Medicaid made available large amounts of matching funds for the ever hard-pressed states if they provided certain services. While coverage for patients in state mental hospitals was limited to those under 21 and over 65 in need of active medical care for a physical ailment, nursing home requirements under Medicaid were more flexible.

The growing proprietary nursing home industry could absorb many "de-institutionalized patients" and be reimbursed by Medicaid. The states, in turn, could receive matching funds, thereby easing fiscal problems. Thus began the great surge of "deinstitutionalization" of the late 1960s and early 1970s. Available data help to illustrate the trend. The resident population of state mental hospitals in the United States dropped by half—from 490,000 in 1964 to 249,000 in 1973.[38] The population in nursing homes (not all of these were from mental hospitals) grew by 53 percent from 1963 to 1973, reaching one million.[39] An important reason for the ability to get the patients out of mental hospitals was the availability of nursing homes and the federal funds to help pay for them.

The deinstitutionalization activity eventually became known as "dumping"; patients were "dumped" into nursing homes or into boarding houses. In many cases, elderly, long-stay patients were simply shifted from the mental hospital to the nursing home, for they were unable to cope in the community. Their diagnoses were mostly "brain syndromes" and psychoses, and they were not expected to improve. Over half of all nursing home patients are said to be suffering from some kind of mental disorder, yet the vast majority of nursing homes are ill equipped to care for or treat these patients.[40] In part, at least, this trend toward moving people from state hospitals to nursing homes was seen as the only way to "deinstitutionalize" because of the lack of services in the community.[41]

Problems caused by the lack of services became evident as the number of readmissions to psychiatric hospitals rose to 54 percent of total admissions in 1972.[42]. The community mental health centers were established in 1963 to help, but they did not really reach former mental hospital populations. In communities everywhere, there were insufficient mental health and related services to help these people, and there has as yet been no large-scale funding for them.

The deinstitutionalization impetus also affected the mentally retarded, and to a substantial extent, they met with the same problem. But the advocates and families of the mentally retarded were alert and through persuasion, pressure, and litigation have enlisted the services of school systems, the federal government (Medicaid, SSI), and other community organizations to assist them. A large portion of SSI federal payments and state supplements for congregate care now goes to the mentally retarded in domiciliary care settings; in some states over half of these residents are retarded.[43]

The Role of Institutions

The nursing home, the psychiatric hospital, and the institution for the mentally retarded can all be expected to remain; it would not be desirable to see them disappear altogether, though they will undoubtedly change. There will continue to be people with care needs which can only be met by institutions; 24-hour surveillance, round-the-clock nursing services, and certain rehabilitation services cannot easily or economically be provided in the home. As a means of protecting people from society, people from themselves, and society from people, there is a continuing need for institutions.

What is needed is not one or another of a variety of separate services and settings, but a spectrum of services that work together or in logical progression to assist the client. Thus, the institution would ideally be a part of the community, either providing some services to the community, or making use of community resources instead of attempting to duplicate them.

The extent of actual need for institutions will be seen only after the full range of essential community services is in place and is widely used by the chronically ill and impaired. Certainly the need for a continued high rate of nursing home construction will have to be closely examined and the need for inpatient beds will have to be considered in conjunction with other service needs and availability. At some point funding will have to be diverted from institutions to expanded community services.

LONG-TERM CARE FINANCING PROGRAMS AND THE PROBLEM OF INTERPROGRAM COORDINATION

Throughout this chapter, we have emphasized the importance of service effectiveness and the need for greater coordination among the programs designed to meet the needs of the long-term care population. It has become apparent that many public programs do not work either economically, appropriately, or effectively to the benefit of the populations at risk. Two of the major reasons for these shortcomings are an inflexible and irrelevant program structure and the lack of a rationally integrated system of programs. Before we examine these problems in greater detail, however, we will survey the programs that presently provide services and benefits to the populations at risk.

Medicaid (Title XIX of the Social Security Act)

Medicaid finances a comprehensive range of health and medical services, some required and some at state discretion. The services described below are in addition to physician, inpatient hospital, clinic, and other routine medical services. It is the largest source of funding and reimbursement for services to the disabled, impaired, and chronically ill.

Institutional Care Under Medicaid

Most long-term care under Medicaid is currently institutional in nature. Skilled nursing facility (SNF) services are provided for individuals over 21 years of age (optional for the under 21) who need, on a daily basis, SNF or other skilled rehabilitation services, which as a practical matter can only be provided in an SNF on an inpatient basis. Eligibility for SNF care must be certified by a physician and is subject to medical review and utilization review for quality and appropriateness.

Intermediate care facility (ICF) services are optional under Medicaid but are now included in 49 state plans. They are intended to provide health-related care and services to individuals who do not require the degree of care and treatment which a hospital or SNF is designed to provide, but who require care and services above the level of room and board, which as a practical matter can be made available to them only through institutional facilities. Need for ICF care must be certified by a physician and is subject to periodic independent professional review and utilization review.

Services in ICF for the mentally retarded are also optional. Health-related care of persons in public institutions for the mentally retarded and persons with related conditions can be reimbursed by Medicaid. The primary purpose of the institution, or distinct part of it, must be provision of health and rehabilitative services and an active treatment program for the mentally retarded. Precertification of need based on client evaluation is required for Medicaid reimbursement.

Finally, institutions for mental diseases also provide certain long-term care services which may be covered under the Medicaid program. In-patient hospital care for persons under age 21 is required and optional for those over 65 in institutions for mental disease. Regulations stipulate that care received must be of a health nature and ordered by a physician.

Community Care Under Medicaid

Other than the normal health care received by the general Medicaid population, community-based, long-term care services have been quite limited in scope. There are indications, however, that the Medicaid program is beginning to shift its long-term care emphasis more toward these services. Home health services under Medicaid include services of an intermittent nature: skilled nursing; home health aide; physical, occupational, and speech therapies; medical and social services; and medical supplies and equipment. Medicaid always deferred to Medicare regulations, which, thus, governed home health in this program; as a result, the use of and eligibility for services has been severely restricted. Medicaid has

TABLE 2.2

Medicaid Expenditures in Selected Areas, FY 1975
(in millions)

Service	Expenditure
Total, Medicaid	$12,028*
Skilled Nursing Facilities	2,200
Intermediate Care Facilities	1,838
ICF—Mentally Retarded	362
Psychiatric Hospitals	600
Home Health	28

*The federal share is $6,743 million.

Source: Medical Services Administration, Department of Health, Education, and Welfare.

published new regulations of its own that remove Medicare interpretations, clarify eligibility criteria, and broaden the criteria for services.

Personal care services may be provided to a Medicaid recipient in the home if they are not rendered by a family member. The regulation permits health-related services, maintenance, household duties, and assistance in activities of daily living; these services are not necessarily tied to provision of medical services except that they must be supervised by a registered professional nurse and ordered by a physician. Only seven or eight states currently make use of this provision.

Day care services for adults have been studied by the Medicaid program for over five years. There is no specific provision for reimbursement of any variant of day services, but Medicaid has funded studies and contributed to demonstrations of several types of day services. On January 22, 1976, the Medical Services Administration (MSA) issued an information memorandum to state Medicaid agencies defining such services and outlining permissible methods of reimbursement.[44] Two types of services are discussed in this memorandum: the day hospital, providing all medical, diagnostic, rehabilitative, and other services with the exception of bed and full board normally provided in an inpatient hospital; and day treatment, which includes therapeutic services and other basic services, on a lesser plane than the day hospital.

Medicare (Title XVIII of the Social Security Act)

Medicare provides some of the types of services applicable to long-term care; they are prevented by statute and regulation from being long-term. In addition to hospital and physician services, Medicare provides skilled nursing facility (SNF) services on a posthospital, semiacute care basis up to 100 days for each spell of illness. SNFs are defined in the same way under Medicare and Medicaid, although eligibility for this "extended care" is defined differently. The reason for SNF placement must be the same reason as the hospitalization, and the patient must need active skilled nusing care or rehabilitative care on a daily basis. Coinsurance is $9 per day after the first 20 days. Inpatient care in psychiatric hospitals (up to 90 days for each spell of illness with a 190 day lifetime limit) is also reimbursable for patients who meet stringent medical care need requirements.

Home health services are provided under Medicare Part A (hospital insurance) and Part B (supplemental medical insurance). Part A requires a prior hospitalization of at least three days for the same condition for which home health services are needed (condition-related requirements). Part B contains no prior hospitalization requirements, but otherwise the eligibility requirements are the same: the patient must be homebound and be certified by a physician to need skilled nursing care, physical therapy, or speech therapy. Medicare's home health provider definition requires the provider to be a public or private nonprofit agency, which is primarily engaged in providing skilled nursing and other therapeutic services. Proprietary agencies are eligible provided they meet state licensure requirements, which exist in only 16 states, thus limiting the proprietaries to those states. The regulations thus preclude a broad-based health care provider such as a community health center or a health maintenance organization (HMO) from receiving Medicare (or Medicaid, until new regulations are issued) reimbursement for home health services unless they establish a separate administrative mechanism.[45]

Social Services (Title XX of the Social Security Act)

Major problems in assuring availability of social services are the $2.5 billion federal ceiling and the elimination of state maintenance of effort requirements. Funds are distributed on a block grant basis to states, which must then publish their plans for spending the money. All income groups are eligible for service, though at least 50 percent must be low income.

A wide variety of services is available for the states to choose from. The social services have traditionally been provided largely to families with children, but there is now a requirement that at least three services be made available to SSI recipients.

TABLE 2.3

Medicare Expenditures, FY 1975
(in millions)

	HI[a]	SMI[b]	Total
Persons Enrolled			
Aged	21.6	21.5	
Disabled	2.1	1.8	
Received Services			
Aged	4.9	11.2	
Disabled	.6	1.4	
Benefits			
Inpatient Hospital			
Aged	$9,033		$9,033
Disabled	921		921
Skilled Nursing Facility			
Aged	259		259
Disabled	8		8
Home Health Services			
Aged	123	$ 46	169
Disabled	9	5	14
Physician Services			
Aged		2,805	2,805
Disabled		221	221
Outpatient Services			
Aged		402	402
Disabled		198	198
Other Services			
Aged		82	82
Disabled		6	6
Total Medicare	$10,353	$3,765	$14,118

[a]Hospital Insurance.
[b]Supplementary Medical Insurance.
Source: U.S. Office of Management and Budget, *The Budget of the United States Government, FY 1977, Appendix* (Washington, D.C.: Government Printing Office, 1976), pp. 374–75.

TABLE 2.4

Social Services Program Expenditures, FY 1975
(in thousands)

Total Costs	$2,622,364
Federal Share (Total)	1,962,573
Day Care	486,718
Foster Care	264,947
Services to the Mentally Retarded	249,247
Drug Abuse/Alcoholism Services	92,241
Family Planning	43,177
In-Home Services	284,000
All Other (Protective, information, and so on)	542,243

Source: U.S. Office of Management and Budget, *The Budget of the United States Government, FY 1977, Appendix* (Washington, D.C.: Government Printing Office, 1976), p.361.

Title XX services are intended to achieve or maintain independence and prevent inappropriate institutionalization by providing community-based care, in addition to several other goals outlined in the legislation. Services for the impaired and disabled that could be provided include homemaker and chore services, congregate meals, adult day care, adult foster family supervision, home health services, home management, protective services, respite care, mental health services, sheltered workshops, transportation, and many more. Table 2.4 provides a rough breakdown of social services expenditures.

Supplemental Security Income (SSI, Title XVI of the Social Security Act)

Under the SSI program, the aged, blind, and disabled receive a minimum monthly benefit of $157 from the federal government. State supplementation is required for those persons whose previous public assistance payments were higher than the SSI payment; supplementation is optional for all other recipients. States may supplement payments to allow the purchase of congregate care or personal care.

Community Mental Health Centers Program (CMHC)

This program is included as a possibility for the future more than a present solution. Only about 500 federal supported CMHCs have been developed for the entire country; they currently serve a very small proportion of chronic and aged patients, concentrating on persons who have never been institutionalized and who need less intensive and varied services of shorter duration.

The Community Mental Health Centers Act of 1973 authorized construction and staffing grants for the development and delivery of comprehensive mental health services at the local level. The centers are required to offer a range of services, including 24-hour inpatient care, outpatient care, partial hospitalization (day, night, weekend), around-the-clock emergency services, and consultation and education services to community agencies and professional personnel.

The 1975 version of the CMHC Act reflected congressional concern about the narrowness of the population types being served, the publicity for the plight of deinstitutionalized chronic mental patients, and the need for noninstitutional community alternatives. The CMHCs are now required to broaden their scope to serve the chronic patient and the deinstitutionalized patient, to provide halfway house services, screening for service needs, and follow-up services, and to provide more service to the aged.

Vocational Rehabilitation (VR)

Vocational Rehabilitation is a state-federal formula grant program to provide vocational rehabilitation services to physically and mentally disabled persons in order to prepare them for work. A comprehensive range of services is provided to meet this objective: evaluation, counseling, placement, training, physical and mental restoration services, transportation, and many others. The VR program may also pay for hospitalization, convalescent or nursing home care, prosthetic, orthotic, or other assistant devices. Vehicles may be purchased and specially outfitted, and interpreter services for the deaf, attendant services, and education may also be paid for.

Developmental Disabilities (DD)

This program is still very small and is essentially one of resource development, designed to strengthen existing services and provide new services to persons with mental retardation, cerebral palsy, epilepsy, and other neurological conditions. Financial assistance is provided to state agencies for planning, construction, administration, and services or facilities for the developmentally disabled.

Veterans Administration Programs

The VA provides a substantial amount of institutional long-term care, as well as some other relevant services. Eligibility for health services is granted to veterans with service-connected disabilities and to indigent veterans. VA hospitals provide inpatient care, other than surgical or psychiatric, for both short- and long-term patients. These patients are classed as medical bed-care patients, needing a physician's care and treatment daily; and skilled nursing care patients, needing skilled nursing care but not necessarily close medical supervision. There is also a category for patients requiring psychiatric bed care.

In addition to its hospitals, the VA operates or contracts with 18 domiciliary care facilities and nursing homes that provide nursing care, domiciliary care, and social services such as alcoholism rehabilitation, as well as halfway houses for psychiatric patients being returned to the community. The maximum length of stay in nursing homes is six months, except for veterans whose hospitalization was for a service-connected disability.

Traditionally, VA services have been provided in institutions, and it is proving difficult to change that. There is, however, a small hospital-based home care program. In 1973, 8,000 home health visits were made; this is a very small number considering several visits were made to each patient.

The VA finances an aid and attendance program in addition to its health services. Monthly benefits, supplemental to regular benefits, are supplied to housebound and bedbound veterans for use in purchasing "aid and attendance" service. Eligibility for aid and attendance is based on physical or mental disability, which must be certified by the appropriate medical personnel. For those receiving compensation for service-connected disabilities (nonincome-related), there are complicated statutory criteria to determine the amount of the aid and attendance payment; compensation benefits can reach substantial amounts. The program provides the individual in need of attendance with the cash to pay a family member or someone who is willing to provide the service. It is not known what effect the payment has on the recipient, as there are no follow-up or evaluation analyses available to determine the impact or use of the funds.

Housing

Housing is not normally considered to be a part of long-term care, but it should be, for adequate and decent housing is essential to the successful care of a person at home. Congregate housing and special purpose housing for the elderly and handicapped are instrumental in long-term care, and should become even more so.

The Department of Housing and Urban Development does not provide services in the housing it funds (though it can provide space for them), but it does fund special purpose housing for the elderly and the handicapped.

Barriers to Program and Service Coordination

Fragmentation of Service Efforts:

The separation of health from social and economic services in public programs has serious consequences for those in need of long-term care. In spite of the demonstrated overlap between health and social service needs (such as personal care), the Medicaid and Social Services programs do not mesh at all. Even though the two programs used to be administered by the same agency, they never worked closely together. Many individuals argue that Medicaid is a health financing program, not a service program like Title XX, and that, in keeping with this orientation, it draws a line at certain "social" services, in part through its ties with Medicare regulations.

This split is exacerbated by the fact that Medicaid has continued to provide most long-term care within an institutional setting; home health care, a service that under Medicaid must be provided by states, used less than .1 percent of the Medicaid budget in Fiscal Year (FY) 1976. A former commissioner of Medicaid has written that "for the elderly, especially, the integration of health and social services at the local level must be encouraged through the removal of financial incentives to institutionalize people."[46]

States can receive Medicaid reimbursement only for what are recognized as health services; it is sometimes possible under Medicaid, though difficult, to provide personal care services in the home (New York has a caseload of 30,000), and only eight states use this option. The Social Services program can provide similar services, but the eligibility criteria differ.

The effect of these structural constraints is naturally felt most deeply at the local levels, where considerable juggling of programs and funds may be necessary to get needed services to the client. A good example is homemaker service, which may only be provided through Medicaid along with other services as prescribed by a physician; under Title XX the same service must be ordered by a social service worker using different criteria. Either the patient or, more rarely, his representative must cull various programs to find a useful service, then cope with differing entry requirements. To avoid these problems, many providers and clients simply give up on the publicly financed community care system and prescribe institutional care, which will be reimbursed by Medicaid for services the program would not pay for in the community.

Lack of authority to order services, or power to obtain interagency cooperation, has hampered many coordination efforts, so that some local agencies prefer to provide all necessary services to a group of clients defined geographically, by condition or by age. This method obviates the need for coordination, but may encourage fragmentation of services, albeit along different lines than before. It also clouds the need to develop additional community resources to be used by all inhabitants who need them, regardless of their group identification. The question is whether to build a new structure on top of a system of fragmented services and competing agencies, or whether it is possible to rearrange services and reorient the programs—an admittedly difficult task.

Level of Care Barriers to Coordination

A further disincentive to effective, appropriate, and coordinated care is the establishment of various "levels of care" both in and out of institutions. The problems of home care described above should also be considered in this context. For example, the Medicare law fails to provide many needed community services either on a long-term or short-term basis because it requires the evidence of an acute condition for which skilled professional care is needed. Many people do need this type of care for a posthospital or other acute episode, but many who need home health services cannot obtain them through Medicare.

Medicaid has, by law and regulation, established levels of institutional care into which the patient must fit, rather than having services tailored to his needs. Skilled nursing homes serve one level and intermediate care facilities another. Patients whose conditions fluctuate must physically move back and forth among facilities if they are not in one that is certified for both levels. Since the conditions of the chronically ill often do fluctuate, this level of care requirement poses serious problems to the patient. The problem also extends to the mentally retarded in ICFs, for they must be, according to the regulations, in a health-related part of the facility in order to receive Medicaid reimbursement. This encourages distortion in the services claimed by the providers in order to gain the Medicaid reimbursement; it is presumably condoned by states in need of federal funds.

These levels of care exist primarily to aid in the establishment of per diem reimbursement rates and they discourage care based on needs of the patient. They allow decisions about the life and care of the patient to be made by third party payors and reimbursement regulations.

Living Arrangements

Individual choice of living arrangements and care has been affected by discontinuities in definitions between Medicaid and SSI. A major unresolved issue is what types of living settings are reimbursable under each program. Medicaid pays for health and health-related care in various institutions, including intermediate care facilities. Current Medicaid ICF regulations spell out a broad range of health, personal care, and therapeutic services, which, while not essential in every facility, have to be made available to any patient in need of them. In the past, intermediate care facilities have varied greatly among the states; some facilities have provided only the "basics" while others, established as independent sections within skilled nursing facilities, offer fairly sophisticated care. The regulations issued in 1974 and the Medicaid program's subsequent interpretation of them did little to clarify the meaning and requirements of ICFs. States remain uncertain about the kind of ICF expected by HEW, or how HEW will choose to enforce regulations.

Problems of definition have also arisen in connection with care financed through SSI. Under this program, the states have the option to supplement the federal cash benefit. One of the prime areas for optional state supplementation is the financing of living arrangements—especially protection or congregate living and domiciliary care. Thus, many SSI recipients, ranging from the aged and frail to the mentally retarded or mentally ill, receive extra monthly allowances to enable them to pay for congregate care or similar care as defined by the state. What constitutes congregate care for reimbursement purposes has never been made entirely clear, however. It is intended to be more than room and board, but it does not usually encompass health care. The lack of a specific definition led to certain complications with the passage of Public Law 92-603.

Section 1616e of this law, passed in 1972, enjoined the SSI program from using federal cash assistance to pay for institutional care that could be covered by the Medicaid program. The law required dollar-for-dollar reductions of federal SSI funds for every dollar of state supplementation going to support people in institutions that are or could be certified under Medicaid. The intent expressed by the Senate Finance Committee was to prevent substandard nursing homes (which did not or could not meet Medicaid standards) from remaining in operation by receiving SSI payments from individual recipients.[47]

This ruling was felt to be unfair since it penalized the individual for facility shortcomings, and unenforceable because of definitional problems. The inability to draw clear distinctions between a congregate care institution and one that provides "medical or remedial" services made the provision impossible to enforce. In addition, it proved difficult to draw a clear line between a Medicaid-defined intermediate care facility and an SSI facility. The federal government, lacking any firm guidelines, could not readily identify those facilities that offered "medical or remedial" care or those SSI recipients living in them.

In 1976, an attempt to modify or repeal Section 1616e resulted in a requirement that states establish standards for institutions in which a substantial number of SSI recipients reside or are likely to reside. The requirement for reducing the federal SSI benefit to residents of facilities providing medical or remedial care remains.

The attempt to draw rigid lines between SSI-type congregate care facilities and Medicaid facilities results in an artificial dichotomy between "medical" and "social" care. What counts in this type of system is the payment source and program definition rather than the actual state and need of the individual.

Since much nonmedical long-term care occurs in congregate, domiciliary, and personal care facilities, it is clear that SSI is in reality a substantial contributor to such care. The problem of what standards, if any, should be imposed on these facilities, and by whom, has not been satisfactorily resolved. Clearly, many persons in these facilities need more mental or physical care than they receive; how these services should be provided has not been decided. Physical and safety standards are often unenforced, resulting in very bad living conditions.[48] These are issues that will have to be resolved in the future if congregate care is to be effective, decent, and scandal-free. At the present time, it seems that all levels of government are unsure of their responsibilities here, a situation which can result in lack of focus and authority.

AMBULATORY CHRONIC CARE SERVICE PROPOSAL

It is clear that something must be done to improve the delivery of servics of all kinds to the long-term ill and impaired. The fragmentation and uneven distribution of services among people, the lopsided incentives for intitutionalizing, and the poor quality of medical and health care in and out of institutions dictate the need for certain changes. Coordination, assessment, prescription, referral, monitoring, and advocacy activities should be a part of any system of care. They are necessary if we are to see that people receive services that are appropriate to their circumstances.

Simultaneously with current efforts to upgrade institutional services, it is necessary to develop community resources and reduce the almost total reliance on institutions to meet the need for long-term care. Community service programs offer excellent laboratories for experiementation and reform in the provision of long-term care.

A program designed to provide coordinated health and related services to a chronically ill and impaired population should include a set of governing principles:

1. Long-term care is ambulatory care far more than it is an institutional service.

2. Health care of the chronically ill and impaired should be treated in the context of general medical and health care, not as a separate service.

3. The setting and method of delivery of services should fluctuate in accordance with individual requirements.

4. There should be balanced incentives to use community or institutional services (lack of bias) in order to ensure the appropriateness of services received.

5. The community nature of residential facilities should be maintained as much as possible, instead of creating new categories of institutions.

6. Programs and services must be effectively integrated at the client level.

7. Services should be oriented to "living," rather than patienthood.

8. Services must be designed to permit people to live in maximum independence.

9. Existing legislative authorities and constraints should be adapted as much as possible to more flexible use, absent total program revisions.

Program Structure

The Ambulatory Chronic Care Service (ACCS)

At the local, or client level, an agency would be established to exercise these following functions: client assessment (evaluation/diagnosis), prescription, referral, monitoring of client, follow-up, and representation/mediation. The agency would serve as a coordination and assessment agent to its clientele, and would be responsible for seeing that the necessary services are provided to the client, and would assist in matters of program eligibility, finances, and reimbursement. The client would be free to refuse or make changes in services.

Depending upon the model chosen—localities should be allowed to choose among several workable ones—the agency, in addition to providing the assessment and service coordination, would enter into agreements or contracts for services on behalf of the client, in some cases purchasing services with funds set aside for such purposes.

Eligible Populations

All persons eligible for public programs who are aged or disabled would automatically be eligible for assessment/coordination functions at the Ambulatory Chronic Care Service. Medicare and Medicaid eligibles, Social Security and SSI recipients, former mental hospital patients, and former residents of institutions for the retarded would be among those eligible, but the agency should also serve broader groups.

All persons with disabilities, chronic illnesses, and multiple service needs should be eligible for most of the services of the agency, regardless of their income. These people might pay for their own assessment, or be assisted by general funds for the purpose. It is not only the extremely poor who need assistance in coordinating service packages for themselves; although the financially independent might constitute a minority, they should be included. The reimbursement of services for these groups would continue to be out-of-pocket except for what is paid by health insurance or other means.

Service Structure

While only in rare circumstances would the Ambulatory Chronic Care Service actually provide services, it would be responsible for referral to and monitoring of many services. These services would continue to be financed by existing public and private programs.

In the area of health services, acute hospital, extended care, and skilled nursing facility care would remain similar to Medicare-Medicaid, but with no prior hospitalization requirement. Skilled nursing facility care needed over a long period would be financed through a special Medicaid benefit, or through a catastrophic health insurance benefit. Intermediate care for those requiring care in an institution would be reimbursed as a special Medicaid benefit. The ICF facility should be used only if it is impossible to meet the patient's needs in another setting and if the need is certified by the Ambulatory Chronic Care Service. All other health care, whether needed on a long- or short-term basis, would be provided through normal financing and delivery systems: physician services, other medical and health services, medically oriented rehabilitation, day hospital, and day health clinics.

Medicare, Medicaid, and Social Services funds would finance home health services. Such services would be substantially more important than they are now under these programs. The expansion of homemaker-home health aid and personal care services would help to reduce institutions' admissions.

Eligibility criteria would also undergo some changes. Client eligibility criteria would be broadened to allow therapeutic, maintenance, and preventive care in addition to acute care. Provider eligibility criteria would be changed to allow broad health care providers such as community health centers or HMOs to establish home health services.

Residences for recipients would include congregate care facilities, group homes, halfway houses, and other places which do not themselves provide health services but whose residents need health care brought to them.

Medicaid long-term institutional benefits would be retained for the mentally retarded and mentally ill to the extent necessary, based on the criteria outlined for the ICFs.

Social Services

The Social Services program (Title XX) and related programs at the state and local level would provide supportive services to allow the client to remain in the most independent setting. Social services would complement health and medical services, or would be provided as personal maintenance services whether or not health services are needed. Homemaker, transportation, adult day center, personal care, meals on wheels and the Administration on Aging's nutrition program, and other services would be provided. The Area Agencies on Aging could assist in coordinating related services.

To ensure availability of social services to the ACCS population, a portion of Title XX program funds would have to be pledged to that group.

Supplemental Security Income (SSI)

The SSI statute and regulations would be modified to allow the cash payment to continue under certain conditions for a specified duration while the recipient is in a hospital, SNF, or ICF. The continuation of payment (which must now be terminated if the patient remains in a Medicaid facility for the better part of a month) would occur if the patient's evaluation showed a likelihood of return to the community after a certain period, for example six months. This would help protect the person's residence by allowing rent or mortgage payments to continue.

Housing Programs

Housing must be brought into the service picture in order for a community care system to function well. Adequate housing is a major aspect of community long-term care, but without services attached or in some other way available, housing alone can do little for the seriously impaired person. HEW and the Department of Housing and Urban Development (HUD) would seek ways to cooperate and coordinate the operation of their programs, with the ACCS playing a role at the local level. Sheltered housing construction and ongoing financing should be the goals of such cooperation.

Program Financing and Cost Issues

As stated above, most services would continue to be financed by the same programs and in a similar way, unless the general financing structure changed to or from an open-ended program structure or formula grants. If prospective budgeting is found to be a workable method of keeping track of and controlling costs, the ACCS program could be funded in this way, and through several different programs. This in itself would require coordination at the federal level. In addition, current proposals for incentive reimbursement need to be examined to determine their efficacy in controlling costs and quality of services. Both the ACCS and the providers will have to be reimbursed in ways that are different from current practices.

Methods of funding the Amubulatory Chronic Care Service would depend on the organizational scheme chosen, but whatever the method, it must be adequate to develop the capacity of the service. Some administrative funds would come from Medicare and Medicaid, and from Social Services and other programs. Some method of capitation payments could be worked out, for the agency would have a fairly predictable caseload when fully operational. Development and start-up funds would be made available through various federal, state, and local sources, and from private ones as appropriate.

The financing of the actual health and related services would be left as in current programs described above, pending overall reform of these programs. Some incentives will have to be built in to encourage less reliance on institutional care, and more on community services. This means also that the power of the nursing home interests versus the home health agencies and other local providers must be brought into balance so that both have relatively equal influence over allocation decisions and ACCS activities. Otherwise, the same referral process and distortions which now exist will continue.

The Federal Role

There would be a need for authority at the top if a coordination program were to function. There must be a single authority in HEW charged with coordinating and assisting the programs, setting and monitoring standards, and working with other agencies on financing and service issues. The federal government would be responsible for collecting and disseminating knowledge of workable models and activities and would assist in resource development efforts.

Funding and guidance will probably be needed to spur development of more and different community services. Long-term care planning authorities at the federal and local levels must be encouraged to evaluate and enforce priorities between community and institutional service development, and to help integrate chronic care services into the mainstream of health care, while at the same time maintaining a perspective that is wider than health care.

The federal government would undertake data collection of sufficient scope to enable evaluation of program effectiveness. This would consist of routine data collection and survey activities. In addition, the federal government must play an instrumental role in the development, testing, and implementation of better performance standards by which to judge *quality* as well as quantity of services. Finally, the federal government should continue research into coordination and assessment models (in terms of tools and effectiveness) and into service effectiveness, quality, costs, and outcomes.

The State Role

Just as there would be a central coordinative role at the federal level, there would be a similar function within the state government. The states would set up organizations to oversee development and funding of the local ACCS, to monitor performance, designate service areas, certify services, and set and fund the service budgets. The states would also be responsible for maintaining standards of quality care rendered by all providers of services, from nursing homes to congregate living settings. State activities in this area would be based on quality standards designed to assess clients as well as facilities. ACCS efficiency and effectiveness would be included in assessment of quality. In resource development, information dissemination, and data collection, the states would somewhat parallel the federal activities.

Reimbursement of ACCS and provider services should rest at the state rather than the local level. Reimbursement methods need reanalysis to assure that they purchase services of sufficient quality without breaking budgets. Reimbursement incentives should also be used to foster the use of community services instead of institutional care as much as is appropriate.

The Local Role

Local community organizations would be responsible for forming the Ambulatory Chronic Care Services, and with state assistance would work out interagency contracts or other service agreements. Localities would decide how many ACCS agencies they need and establish catchment areas to be served by them, if more than one is necessary.

The local community would identify resource needs and would then develop those resources with the help of federal and state governments. The ACCS would also assist the federal and state powers in the enforcement and monitoring of standards and might assume the responsibility of validating state findings. The ACCS must be kept informed of all deficiencies and ratings of facilities and services in the area, to enable them to make use of the highest quality services within budget constraints.

The ACCS and community service agencies would be responsible for developing prospective budgets to be submitted to the state, and for maintaining data and accounting systems.

Conclusion

A number of options for policy reform have been discussed in Congress, the executive branch of government, the universities, and the public sphere. Some of the options call for modest changes in specific health benefits; others, for large-scale reform in program organization. The ACCS proposal differs from many of these in the sense that it is, at least in part, a generic proposal; it is intended to set forth certain principles that should govern the formulation of any long-term care policy. The proposal does include a number of specific directives, and it entails the creation of an assessment and coordination function at the community level. In addition, however, it defines certain objectives or "conditions" that a long-term care program should meet. The policymakers may decide upon any one of a number of organizational models, but whatever their choice, they must bear in mind the necessity of making long-term care a health-oriented rather than a sickness-oriented system. Measures which would tend to isolate the chronically ill or impaired from the community or to isolate the health care needs of this population from their social and economic needs are inappropriate. The programs which should be designed and funded are those which would enable the individual to live as independently as possible, in the most normative environment possible.

NOTES

1. U.S., Department of Health, Education, and Welfare, Public Health Service, *Health, United States, 1975*, Pubn. no. (HRA) 76-1232 (1976), p. 195.

2. See Saad Z. Nagi, *An Epidemiology of Disability among Adults in the United States* (Columbus: Mershon Center, Ohio State University, 1975), pp. 13, 28.

3. U.S., Congress, Senate, Special Committee on Aging, Subcommittee on Long-Term Care, *Hearing on Trends in Long-Term Care, Part 14*, 92nd Cong., 1st sess., 1971, pp. 1373–1419. Statement of Lionel Z. Cosin.

4. Herman B. Brotman, "The Fastest Growing Minority: The Aging," *American Journal of Public Health* 64, no. 3 (1974), 249–52.

5. U.S., Department of Health, Education, and Welfare, *Health, United States, 1975*, p. 255; and Ethel Shanas, "Measuring the Home Health Needs of the Aged in Five Countries," *Journal of Gerontology* 26, no. 1 (1971), p. 38.

6. U.S., Department of Health, Education, and Welfare, Public Health Service, "Changes in the Age, Sex, and Diagnostic Composition of the Resident Population of State and County Mental Hospitals, U.S., 1964–1973," *Statistical Note 112*, DHEW Pubn. no. (ADM) 75-158 (1975), pp. 6–7.

7. U.S., Department of Health, Education, and Welfare, National Center for Health Statistics, *Chronic Conditions and Impairments of Nursing Home Residents: U.S., 1969* (1973), p. 24.

8. U.S., HEW, NCHS, *Chronic Conditions*, p. 23.

9. Brotman, *The Fastest Growing Minority*, p. 251.

10. New York, State Department of Health, "The Resident-Patient Profile," by Amalia P. Crago, mimeographed (1970), p. 9.

11. Murray Tucker, *Background and Analysis: Long-Term Care for the Mentally Retarded* (Washington, D.C.: The Urban Institute, 1975), p. 4.

12. Ibid., p. 5.

13. U.S., Department of Health, Education, and Welfare, *Mental Retardation Sourcebook* (1974), p. 71.

14. U.S., Department of Health, Education, and Welfare, National Institute of Mental Health, "The Severely Mentally Disordered," by Valerie J. Bradley for use of The White House Conference for Handicapped Individuals (1976), p. 15.

15. Nagi, *An Epidemiology of Disability*, p. 17.

16. Margaret Blenkner, Martin Bloom, and Margaret Nielson, "A Research and Demonstration Project on Protective Services," *Social Casework* 52, no. 8 (1971), 483–99.

17. U.S., Department of Health, Education, and Welfare, Public Health Service, "State and Regional Distribution of Psychiatric Beds in 1974," *Statistical Note 118*, DHEW Pubn. no. (ADM) 75-158 (1975), p. 3.

18. U.S., Department of Health, Education, and Welfare, Public Health Service, "Changes," *Statistical Note 112*, DHEW Pubn. no. (ADM) 75-158 (1975), p. 9.

19. U.S., HEW, NIMH, "The Severely Mentally Disordered," p. 12.

20. U.S., Department of Health, Education, and Welfare, National Institute of Mental Health, *Halfway Houses Serving the Mentally Ill and Alcoholics, U.S., 1973*, DHEW Pubn. no. (ADM) 76-264 (1975), p. 12.

21. Irving R. Rutman, "Adequate Residential and Community-Based Programs for the Mentally Disabled" (Philadelphia: Horizon House Institute for Research and Development, 1976), pp. 7–8. (Paper prepared for The White House Conference on Handicapped Individuals.)

22. U.S., HEW, NIMH, "The Severely Mentally Disordered," pp. 19–20.

23. Robert Morris, Ilana Lescohier, and Ann Withorn, *Social Service Delivery Systems: Attempts to Alter Local Patterns, 1970–1974* (Waltham, Mass.: Brandeis University, 1975), p. 60.

24. U.S., Department of Health, Education, and Welfare, *Final Report of Service Integration for Deinstitutionalization*, RSA Grant No. 15-P-55896/3-02, p. 25.

25. William G. Bell, "Community Care for the Elderly, An Alternative to Institutionalization," *The Gerontologist* 13, no. 3, part 1 (1973), 349–54.

26. U.S., Department of Health, Education, and Welfare, General Accounting Office. *Problems in Providing Proper Care to Medicaid and Medicare Patients in Skilled Nursing Homes* (1971), pp. 1–49.

27. U.S., Department of Health, Education, and Welfare, National Center for Health Statistics, *Characteristics of Patients in Nursing and Person Care Homes* (1969), p. 10.

28. Burton Dunlop, *Draft Report on an Informal Look at the Long-Term Care Assessment-Placement Process: Present Problems and Future Prospects* (Washington, D.C.: The Urban Institute, 1975), pp. 6–8.

29. Ibid., pp. 13–14.

30. U.S., Congress, Senate, Special Committee on Aging, *Adult Day Facilities for Treatment, Health Care, and Related Services*, by Brahna Trager, 94th Cong., 2d sess., 1976, p. 4.

31. U.S., Congress, Senate, *Home Health Services in the United States: A Report to the Special Committee on Aging*, by Brahna Trager, 92nd Cong., 2d sess., 1972, p. 5.

32. Robert M. Moroney and Norman R. Kurtz, "The Evolution of Long-Term Care Institutions," in Sylvia Sherwood, ed., *Long-Term Care* (New York: Spectrum Publications Inc., 1975), p. 87.

33. Moroney and Kurtz, "Evolution," pp. 87–88.

34. For detailed reports, see U.S., Congress, Senate, Special Committee on Aging, Subcommittee on Long-Term Care, *Nursing Home Care in the United States: Failure in Public Policy*, Introductory Report and Paper No. 1, 93rd Cong., 2d sess., 1974, pp. 1–241.

35. Texas Department of Mental Health and Mental Retardation, Final Report of the Study of Placement Needs of State Mental Hospital Patients, NIMH Contract No. (ADM) 42-74-81 (OP), by Daniel M. Sheehan and James E. Craft (1974), Table VI, p. 18 (Mimeographed).

36. Robert L. Berg, Francis E. Browning, John G. Hill, and Walter Wenkert, "Assessing the Health Care Needs of the Aged," *Health Services Research*, Spring 1970, 36–59; and John W. Davis and Marilyn J. Gibbin, "An Areawide Examination of Nursing Home Use, Misuse, and Nonuse," *American Journal of Public Health* 61, no. 6 (1971), 1146–55.

37. Texas Department of Mental Health, Table VI, p. 18; Table XII, p. 31; and Table XI, p. 27.

38. U.S., HEW, "Changes," *Statistical Note 112*, p. 6.

39. Urban Institute, *Nursing Home Supplies and Demands, 1964–1974* (Washington: Urban Institute, 1975). Mimeographed.

40. U.S., Department of Health, Education, and Welfare, Office of Nursing Home Affairs, *Long-Term Care Facility Improvement Study*, Introductory Report, Pubn. No. (OS) 76-50021 (July 1975).

41. U.S., Congress, Senate, Special Committee on Aging, *Mental Health Care and the Elderly: Shortcomings in Public Policy*, S. Rept. 38-5960, 92nd Cong., 1st sess., 1971, pp. 1–194.

42. U.S. Department of Health, Education, and Welfare, "Readmissions to Inpatient Sevices of State and County Mental Hospitals, 1972," *Statistical Note 110*, DHEW Pubn. No. (ADM) 75-158 (1974), p. 3.

43. Booz, Allen, and Hamilton, Inc., *Study of the Impact on State Supplementation of SSI Payments for Domiciliary Care on SSI Recipients in Care*, mimeographed (Washington, D.C., June 1975).

44. U.S., Department of Health, Education, and Welfare, Social and Rehabilitation Service, "Reimbursement under Title XIX, Social Security Act, for Services to the Chroni-

cally Ill and Impaired in Alternative Settings," Information Memorandum, SRS-IM-76-3 (MSA), January 22, 1976.

45. U.S., Department of Health, Education, and Welfare, Office of the Assistant Secretary of Planning and Evaluation, *Home Health Care: Development Problems and Potential*, by Marie Callender and Judith LaVor, mimeographed (April 1975); and U.S., Congress, Senate, Special Committee on Aging, *Home Health in the United States*, by *Brahna Trager, 92nd Cong., 2d sess., 1972, pp. 7'9.*

46. U.S., *Department of Health, Education, and Welfare, Medical Services Administration, "The Lessons of Medicaid," by Howard N. Newman, mimeographed (June 1974).*

47. U.S., *Congress, Senate, Committee on Finance, Report on H.R. 1*, S. Rept. 1230, 92nd Cong., 2d sess., 1972, pp. 308–9.

48. U.S., Congress, Senate, Special Committee on Aging, Subcommittee on Long-Term Care, *Nursing Home Care in the U.S.: Failure In Public Policy*, Supporting Paper No. 7, "The Role of Nursing Homes in Caring for Discharged Mental Patients (and the Birth of a For-Profit Boarding Home Industry)," 94th Cong., 2nd sess., 1976, pp. 703–81.

3

OPTIONS FOR FEDERAL FINANCING OF LONG-TERM CARE

Eddie W. Correia

THE EXISTING SYSTEM

Introduction

There are a number of special problems in the public financing of long-term care. The costs of medical care for the chronically ill and impaired continue to increase rapidly, at the same time that changing longevity and birth patterns have caused the population at risk to expand. Expenditures under the Medicaid program—the primary vehicle for federal financing of long-term care at present—have spiraled with the rising costs of institutional care. Despite this large outlay of public funds, considerable dissatisfaction with the quality and availability of care exists.

The lack of a precise definition of "long-term care services" poses additional problems for government financing of long-term care. While health services account for the greatest share of Medicaid expenditures in this area, they represent only one component of comprehensive long-term care. Social and supportive services figure in some way in most conventional definitions of long-term care, and limited coverage for certain services is provided under Medicaid, but policymakers have yet to acknowledge the real importance of these services and to allot to them a sufficient percentage of our public resources. Until agreement is reached on what services constitute, or should constitute, publicly financed long-term care, the extent of government responsibility in this area will remain unclear.

The Medicaid Program

Many of the problems of the long-term care system have been tied to the structure and financing methods of the Medicaid program. Medicaid is administered by the states under federal guidelines. The federal government shares in the cost of a broad range of health and medical services, including physician and inpatient hospital services, care in skilled nursing facilities (SNFs) and intermediate care facilities (ICFs), and some health-related care in institutions for the mentally ill. Coverage for selected home health and community-based services is available, but it is very limited in scope. Some of these services must be provided by the states as a condition of participation in the Medicaid program; other services, such as ICF care and SNF and home health care for persons under 21, are provided at the discretion of the states.

Table 3.1 shows total Medicaid expenditures and expenditures for long-term care services in FY 1976.

Program Deficiencies

The Medicaid program has met with considerable criticism in recent years. One indication of public dissatisfaction with the program is furnished by the numerous proposals for a national health insurance (NHI) plan. The majority of these proposals call for the termination or substantial revision of Medicaid. While the authors of some NHI proposals have chosen to retain the program to finance long-term care, their decision

TABLE 3.1

FY 1976 Medicaid LTC Expenditures

Service	Expenditure (million)	Percent of Total Expenditures
All Services	$13,977	100
Skilled Nursing Facilities	2,549	18.2
Intermediate Care Facilities	2,728	19.5
Home Health Care	129	.9

Source: Medicaid Management Reports, Annual Report, FY 1976, U.S. Department of Health, Education, and Welfare, Medical Services Administration, p. 18.

probably stems more from the difficulty of devising a better system than from a conviction that the current one is particularly effective.

A review of the shortcomings of the Medicaid system becomes the necessary prologue to any recommendations for changing the nature of the federal role in the financing of long-term care. In particular, the personal difficulties that the chronically ill and impaired encounter under the existing system must be taken into consideration in devising alternative means of financing services for this population.

Financial Access to Care:

Not all persons who are in need of some type of long-term care are able to purchase it. The Medicaid and Medicare programs have in particular tended to overlook the needs of a substantial group of persons, mostly persons over 65, whose chronic physical limitations make independent living difficult. This population falls into two major categories—those who are bedfast or essentially totally dependent, and those who are homebound and need help with a limited number of daily tasks and activities, such as preparing meals, eating, bathing, and dressing. While many persons with comparable limitations receive care in skilled nursing homes or intermediate care facilities, millions of bedfast and homebound individuals continue to reside in the community. Various estimates of their numbers are available. The 1966 Social Security Survey of the Disabled found that 4.0 million persons aged 18 to 64 living outside of institutions were confined to their homes or beds.[1] A study of the noninstitutionalized population over 65 years of age estimated that .4 million were bedfast, 1.2 million were housebound, and 1.2 million could move about only with difficulty.[2]

The provision of home health and supportive services would enable these individuals to carry out the daily activities they cannot perform unassisted and would allow them to maintain some level of independent living. Such home health services are, however, extremely restricted under present programs. As indicated in Table 3.1, in fiscal year 1976, the Medicaid program spent a total of only $129 million on home health care—less than 1 percent of total Medicaid expenditures. Moreover, the home health services of both Medicaid and Medicare have historically been directed toward those with short-term illness who require relatively skilled care rather than those with long-term disabilities who require support in the basic tasks of daily living. Medicaid and Medicare tend to exclude a much larger group of persons needing noninstitutional care than they serve. In general, then, limited coverage of noninstitutional services under existing programs represents one of the chief financial barriers to adequate care.

Catastrophic Costs of Care

The Medicaid program provisions for coverage of long-term institutional care tend to impose a drastic financial burden on beneficiaries. To become eligible for Medicaid assistance, persons are required to spend a substantial portion of their income before Medicaid begins to pay for institutional care. Ordinarily, single persons who enter an institution must spend all their income except $25 per month. If one member of a couple enters an institution, the spouse is allowed to retain the state cash assistance payment standard for a single person. Persons receiving Supplemental Security Income payments incur a reduction in cash benefits. A single person receives $25 per month if he or she enters an institution, and a spouse of an inpatient receives the single person's standard.

Inadequate Alternatives to Institutional Care

Many critics of Medicaid have observed that the system has a built-in bias toward institutional care. Because federal financing is largely tied to SNFs and ICFs, the states are discouraged from developing alternatives to institutions. Many forms of community care, for example, cannot be reimbursed under Medicaid.

One consequence of this reimbursement bias is inappropriate placement. Various studies estimate the number of persons inappropriately institutionalized to be from 20 to 80 percent.[3] Unnecessary institutionalization can be costly, debilitating psychologically and physically, and simply a degrading and unhappy experience. While some persons, particularly those who need around-the-clock care, are more efficiently cared for in an institutional setting, many could be deinstitutionalized at a cost saving if appropriate alternative care settings were available.

Inequality Among States

Because of the structure of Medicaid, there is substantial variation in the comprehensiveness of benefits available to the low-income population in each state. SNFs, for example, are required in state Medicaid programs only for persons over 21; only 43 states cover persons under 21. ICFs are not required in any state. While all 50 states provide general ICF care, only 43 provide ICF care for the mentally retarded.[4] In addition, there are variations in income standards for program eligibility.

There is also a substantial variation in expenditures for services from one state to the next. The California and New York Medicaid programs account for 35 percent of total Medicaid expenditures,[5] while only 15 percent of the nation's poor live in those states.[6] Similarly, there is substantial variation in expenditures per eligible person through the Social Services program. In general, the larger states with higher per capita incomes spend more; poorer, less industrialized states spend less.

Poor Quality Standards for Institutional Care

The quality of institutional care for the aged and chronically disabled—whether federally subsidized or not—has been a longstanding concern of the public and Congress. There has been a gradual upgrading of standards for SNFs and ICFs that are eligible for Medicaid vendor payments. Federal enforcement of standards for ICFs began in 1974, and estimates of the capacity of the ICFs to meet federal standards within a reasonable time range widely. In general, federal control over institutional standards is tied to federal expenditures for this type of care. Nevertheless, there have been significant limitations on the practical implications of federal quality standards.

Rapid Increases in Costs

The costs of the Medicaid program have risen substantially over the decade of its existence. Total medical assistance payments were $7.64 billion in FY 1972 and were $14.64 billion in FY 1976[7]—an increase of about 92 percent. Expenditures for ICF care in FY 1973 were approximately $1,162 million and were $2.73 billion in FY 1976.[8] These increases are due in large part to the steadily increasing cost of institutional care. The monthly cost of SNF and ICF care has continued to rise rapidly. The costs of the Medicaid program have also increased because of the federal requirement that ICFs be reimbursed on a reasonable cost basis.

ISSUES IN PROGRAM PLANNING

Certain policy issues must be resolved in formulating new strategies for the federal financing of long-term care. Three of the most significant issues center on the determination of the target population, the role of the states in the administration of a long-term care program, and the nature of federal financing of services.

Allocating Limited Resources to the Needy Population

A comprehensive long-term care program, if extended to serve all income classes and to provide supportive social services furnished on a noninstitutional basis, could entail substantial additional public expenditures. The discussion above suggested there were about 4.0 million persons under 65 and about 1.6 million persons over 65 who were bedfast or confined to their homes and, consequently, in need of supportive social services. As an example of the possible magnitude of costs, providing homemaker services to this population at a cost of only $50 per month would cost $3.36 billion.

In addition to the possible expenditures for noninstitutional care, federal expenditures for institutional care could increase substantially as well. In FY 1976, total national expenditures for nursing home care were $10.6 billion. Public expenditures in the same year were $5.86 billion or about 55 percent of the total.[9] The Medicaid program is currently limited to financing care for the low-income population only, and its provisions require substantial "cost-sharing" from even that population in the form of contributions by patients to the cost of their own care. A decision to expand federal responsibility for long-term care for both the noninstitutionalized and middle-class populations could entail very large additional expenditures. Thus, a major decision will be along what lines to limit any expansion of federal support.

The Role of the States

Policymakers will also have to decide how much latitude the states should have in making use of federal funds. The states already play a major role in administering the Medicaid program; under any new long-term care program, their authority to allocate funds for different services might be extended. In considering this possibility, policymakers will undoubtedly look to the past performance of the states. There has been a great disparity among the states in the types of services offered and in the expenditures per recipient. The states have also differed in the quality standards for institutional care they are willing to tolerate. It is probable that, if left on their own, some states would retain something close to federal standards, while others would tolerate very low levels.

The argument for expanding the state role rests on the assumption that the states are more capable of responding to local circumstances than the federal government. In the past, each state's Medicaid program has been dominated by the restrictions on services mandated by the federal government and the conditions upon which federal financial sharing is contingent. If the states were free to assign funds as they saw fit, they might bring about a more equitable and efficient program of services, tailored to the needs of their individual populations.

The trade-off is apparent. As the states are given more discretion in the use of federal funds, the quality of the services will vary more from state to state. On the other hand, the innovation and responsiveness to local needs will increase. The more the states are limited in discretion, the more uniform the availability and quality of care will be everywhere in the country, and the more likely federal quality standards are to be enforced.

Insurance Financing Versus Fixed Budget Allocation

The third choice that confronts policymakers concerns the appropriate model for financing long-term care. Because long-term care can be defined as a "health" or at least "health-related" service, and because the need of the individual for these services over any given period of time is uncertain, an argument can be made that long-term care services should be financed like acute health services. The appropriate model for the financing of acute medical services is generally considered to be that developed by private health insurance. That system has the following components: (a) a fee for service reimbursement to professional providers, (b) a fixed schedule of covered benefits for which reimbursement can be made, and (c) reimbursement based on a decision by private health providers as to what constitutes "necessary" services. Because the insurance method of financing results in a commitment by the third-party carrier to reimburse for covered services, the budget cannot be prospectively fixed.

The alternative to insurance financing is fixed budget allocations. Expenditures for other government social services are typically made on this basis. Each public program has a fixed budget and must adhere to certain guidelines that define how the budget can be spent. Public social service agencies are charged with allocating the budget.

There are reasons to prefer fixed budget allocation as a means of financing long-term care. First, the demand for long-term care appears to be fairly responsive to price. One study reports the demand for nursing home care has a high price elasticity of demand.[10] Intuitively, it would seem that the demand for certain noninstitutional services, such as homemaker or nutrition services, would be even more price elastic because of the general desirability of these services regardless of illness.

Secondly, there are substantial opportunities to substitute certain types of long-term care services for others. Home health care by relatively unskilled health workers might alleviate the need for nursing home care, and care by relatives might be substituted for care by health workers. Finally, there tends to be a lack of consensus about the "need" for certain services as suggested by the various estimates of the number of persons inappropriately institutionalized.

All these factors point to giving social service agencies greater control over expenditures for long-term care services than is possible under insurance financing. When price elasticity of demand is high, and there is a great opportunity for substitution of less expensive for more expensive services, insurance financing can encourage inefficiency in the way services are utilized. This type of financing involves little or no out-of-pocket cost to consumers, and consumption decisions are typically made by health professionals with no financial stake in limiting the overall cost of the service mix.

FINANCING OPTIONS

Before we outline our own model for the financing of long-term care, we survey the four basic approaches to federal involvement in this area.

The first approach involves cash payments based on disability. This approach provides maximum flexibility and gives the individual a large measure of personal choice. Recipients could take advantage of the widest possible alternatives for meeting their long-term care needs. On the other hand, this system is the most difficult to administer and potentially the most costly. It has the unfortunate tendency to provide a strong incentive for persons to exaggerate their disabilities. In order to provide cash payments adequate to purchase institutional care, very high payments—$400 to $800 per month—would be required. Such a payment to all persons who are good candidates for institutional care, but who are now living outside institutions, would create an enormous financial burden on the program. For these two reasons, the approach is unworkable.

A second approach proposes vendor payments for institutional care. Long-term care services, or at least institutional care, could be financed like acute health services. The cost-sharing would have to be modified somewhat to take account of the fact that a long-term stay in a nursing home takes the place of daily living expenses for food and shelter. However, noninstitutional services, except for a fairly limited home health care benefit, do not lend themselves to an insurance-vendor payment system of financing because of the difficulty of establishing the "need" for such services. Thus, if insurance financing is to be retained, the best approach is a modification of the current Medicaid program—continuation of vendor payments to institutional providers and grants to the states to provide expanded noninstitutional services. This approach has the advantage of ensuring access to institutional services for at least the low-income population; the states would be required to provide individual entitlement to all low-income persons in need of such care. In addition, grants to states for noninstitutional services—small congregate living arrangements, day care, nutrition and homemaker services, and so on—give the states flexibility to create alternatives to institutional care while retaining control over expenditures for these services.

A third alternative is to provide federal grants to states on the basis of per capita income and population. This method of financing would eliminate the matching fund principle that is central to the current Medicaid system. The states would have wide discretion in determining what services would be funded and how the funds should be distributed. The federal government might impose certain constraints on the states' authority; it might dictate, for example, that the funds be used on a particular range of services or require that a minimum portion of grant funds be set aside for the low-income population.

Nevertheless, this approach would give the state governments maximum flexibility. Financing would no longer be tied to institutional care, and the states would have a free hand to research and develop alternatives to institutional care. This option also has the advantage of concentrating responsibility for resource allocation into a single decision-making entity. The states would not have incentives, in the form of federal matching funds tied to institutional care, to maintain inefficient provision of care. Finally, this alternative might result in substantial equality in per capita expenditures from state to state. If grants were provided on a nonmatching basis, using population as a criterion, each state would spend the same amount per capita. If grants were provided on a proportional matching basis, however, the same wide variation in expenditures and quality standards would continue to exist.

However, this approach has two major disadvantages. It terminates individual entitlement; the federal government would have no guarantee that certain persons were receiving the particular services they needed. Secondly, it eliminates federal control of institutional quality standards. Giving states flexibility to spend their grants would also tend to give the states flexibility to spend them for low-quality care.

A variation of the last alternative is to allocate federal grants to local long-term care agencies serving particular regions. This approach could be used to finance long-term care in all settings, or could be limited to non-institutional care only. Grants could be made to private, nonprofit agencies or to local public agencies, or to both.

This approach has the advantage of giving the agency flexibility in allocating benefits and responding to local needs as well as control of expenditures difficult to obtain under an insurance-reimbursement system. In spending federal grants, these long-term care agencies would probably be more accountable to the federal government than the states. It would be politically easier to terminate the grants of an agency that did not adhere to quality standards than to reduce the annual allocations to a state. In addition, these agencies would have less chance to divert grant funds away from the program's intended beneficiaries than would the states, with their wide range of possible uses of grant funds.

One disadvantage of this option is the lack of accountability of these agencies to consumers. They have the same interest in cost-savings as state social service agencies. However, the determination of how well they responded to local needs would rest primarily with the federal government rather than with state officials. An additional disadvantage of this approach is that, historically, grant programs to private, nonprofit agencies have tended to create well-funded elaborate programs in some geographical areas and to leave other areas unserved.

A Model for the Federal Financing of Long-Term Care

The most workable options are a continuation of insurance financing for institutional services with expanded grants for noninstitutional services (option 2) and grants to states (option 3). Much of one's preference between the two depends on the trade-off between uniformity and individual entitlement on the one hand, and flexibility to respond to local needs on the other. From our point of view, option 2 is the most desirable. A fuller description and evaluation of this option follows.

The option has two principal components. First, federal matching funds would continue to be provided to any state that provided a state-administered individual entitlement program for SNF and ICF care. To this extent, the Medicaid program would be continued for these services. However, eligibility requirements and cost-sharing would be uniform in every state, and all states would be required to offer unlimited stays in an SNF and ICF, including ICF care for the mentally retarded, to persons of all ages. In this respect, the option is unlike Medicaid because it eliminates certain discretionary powers of the states.

The second component of the option is a significant expansion of federal matching grants to the states. These supplementary funds could be used only for noninstitutional long-term care, including home health care, day care, and homemaker and transportation services. The funds could not be spent for care in an institutional setting or merely for room and board in a boarding home.

Matching funds for the institutional component of the program would be made on a 60 percent state–40 percent federal basis. On the other hand, matching grants for the noninstitutional component would be made on a 60 percent federal–40 percent state basis. In addition, the concept of individual entitlement for SNF and ICF care would be rigorously maintained so that the states would be required to reimburse for this type of care if a medical determination certified that a patient required this level of care. At the same time, however, the states would have strong financial incentives to provide alternatives to institutional care, and a patient or his family (or some representative) could choose the noninstitutional alternative if available.

Eligibility and Benefits:

All persons needing care would be eligible for long-term SNF and ICF care subject to a cost-sharing requirement. In other words, the categorical and income limitations on Medicaid eligibility would be terminated and replaced by an income-related, cost-sharing arrangement. Each person admitted to a SNF or an ICF would pay cost-sharing based on the following schedule:

Family Group	*Monthly Cost Sharing**
Single Person	30 percent of cost of care plus ⅔ monthly income over SSI benefit payment level; maximum of monthly income minus $50.
Two-Person Family	30 percent of cost of care plus ½ of monthly family income over $250; maximum of monthly income minus $250.
Four-Person Family	30 percent of cost of care plus ⅓ of monthly family income over $500; maximum of monthly income minus $500.

*A ceiling would be placed on maximum payment to an institution to avoid subsidizing very high-cost institutional care.

This cost-sharing is only suggestive. Under these cost-sharing formulas, benefits of the program taper out for a two-person family with an annual income of about $12,000. Cost-sharing can be varied depending on projected program expenditures.

The noninstitutional component of the program would be administered differently. While the proposed increase in federal grants would make comunity and home health services more readily available, there would be no "individual entitlement" for these services. Instead, the states would determine who is eligible to receive services. Persons judged eligible for services would retain their full SSI payment or any state cash supplements if they continued to live in their own homes or in a small group setting.

The exact nature of the "benefits," or services, offered under the program would also be left largely to the states. The states might allot funds to cover care in congregate settings, day care, and home care. Funds could be used for supportive social services to persons in group living settings outside SNFs and ICFS and vendor payments for a "package" of social and remedial services. The states would be limited in their distribution of benefits only to the extent that they could not use funds to cover care in an institutional setting or simple room and board (exclusive of other services).

Costs

The solution of certain problems in the long-term care sector will inevitably require higher federal expenditures than those in the current Medicaid program. As we pointed out in the first section of this chapter, there is a large population now residing outside institutions who require long-term care services. Meeting their needs will place a considerable cost burden on the federal government. In addition, any new financing plan should offer some relief to those Medicaid beneficiaries who are currently forced to make very large out-of-pocket expenditures before Medicaid will begin to cover the costs of institutional care.

Current (FY 1976) federal expenditures under Medicaid for SNF and ICF care are approximately $3.0 billion, or 57 percent of the total.[11] This option calls for reducing the federal share for SNF and ICF care to 40 percent and, in addition, it encourages the states to provide alternatives to institutional care. On the other hand, it reduces cost-sharing so that the public share of costs of care for each person would increase. If it is assumed that the increased cost-sharing and decreased rate of utilization of SNF and ICF care will offset each other, federal expenditures for institutional care under this option would be (40/55) × $3.0 billion or $2.19 billion, a reduction of $.81 billion.

On the other hand, federal expenditures for noninstitutional care will go up. Current federal Medicaid expenditures for home health care are $73 million.[12] In the beginning of the chapter, we reported that there are 4.0 million persons, age 18 to 64, and 1.6 million noninstitutionalized persons who are bedfast or housebound. In addition, a portion of the one million persons who are now in nursing homes will be deinstitutionalized if the states provide noninstitutional alternatives. Based on various studies of "unnecessary institutionalization," 20 percent of this population is a conservative estimate of those who could rely on noninstitutional alternatives. Assuming a 50 percent utilization rate among these groups and an average expenditure of $100 per month per person, total noninstitutional expenditures would be .5 × (4.0 million + 1.6 million + .2 million) × $1,200 or $3.48 billion. The federal share under this option would be 60 percent of this figure or $2.09 billion—substantially above current Medicaid home health expenditures. Thus, federal long-term care (noninstitutional) expenditures would increase by $2.02 billion over Medicaid, and overall long-term care expenditures would increase by $1.21 billion.

Discussion

This approach preserves the advantages of individual entitlement to SNF and ICF care while making cost-sharing and eligibility for this care uniform from state to state. Thus, every person would be guaranteed access to long-term care institutions which meet federal quality standards. In addition, the option limits the 100 percent "spend-down" for the near poor and lower middle-income groups. The cost-sharing scheme is also designed to limit inefficient overutilization of SNF and ICF care by retaining significant cost-sharing; and by relating out-of-pocket costs to the costs of the institution, it encourages persons to choose efficient providers of care.

There would be strong incentives under this option for states to provide care in noninstitutional settings. First, the federal matching rate would be higher for noninstitutional services. Second, SNF and ICF care would be relatively more expensive to the states since cost-sharing would be less than it is now under Medicaid. Third, states will have expanded funds available for use to develop alternatives to institutional care. Since there will be individual entitlement to federally regulated SNF and ICF care, states will have an incentive to attract persons to noninstitutional care, which is both preferable for the individual patient and less expensive to the state.

There are a number of possible problems with this option. First, the institutional component of the program might be so expensive to states that they may choose to rely entirely on grants and simply not offer SNF and ICF care. However, those states that may opt not to offer these benefits (and it seems unlikely for most states because of their heavy institutional burden), even stronger federal incentives might be provided.

While a state may choose to offer SNF and ICF care, it may attempt to direct persons to inferior long-term care alternatives without offering patients a real choice to enter an institution, even if they require that level of care. However, patients should be assured of some representative who will act to enforce their individual entitlement to these institutional benefits. The choice of the noninstitutional alternative would rest with the patient.

A final disadvantage is that the use of matching rates will result in some states taking full advantage of the program while others offer only limited benefits. To some extent, this tendency can be offset by requiring each state to offer uniform services with uniform eligibility requirements. In addition, low-income states could be allowed higher federal matching rates, although the relative institutional and noninstitutional federal matching rates would remain the same.

The Model and Proposals for National Health Insurance

While our model has certain disadvantages, it does address itself to issues that have been largely overlooked by other proposals for reform in the financing of health services. The majority of the proposals for a national health insurance (NHI) program do not incorporate all of the long-term care services now covered under Medicaid into their basic benefit package. Instead, they rely on a number of different approaches intended to provide care to those unable to pay and at the same time, to control expenditures within reasonable bounds. A review of the NHI proposals indicates that the provisions for long-term care services are not always clear; areas of care such as home health or mental health may be overlooked altogether, or the nature and duration of benefits may be left unspecified. A lack of full commitment to the needs of the long-term care population and a certain indirection in meeting these needs characterize many of the NHI proposals.

SNF and ICF care under the NHI proposals are representative of the problem. The typical NHI plan does *not* include unlimited SNF and ICF care in the regular schedule of covered benefits. It relies instead on the continuation of Medicaid to provide financing for extended stays in an SNF or ICF, while offering a limited benefit—of, for example, 100–120 days—in a SNF after a hospital stay. One of the few proposals that departs from the typical NHI plan in this respect is a catastrophic coverage plan providing unlimited stays for all persons in skilled nursing facilities. A large deductible would limit the significance of the SNF benefit for middle-income families, but the deductible for low-income persons would be minimal, virtually eliminating the "spend-down" requirement that currently exists under Medicaid for this group. The plan, although generously conceived, would give rise to certain other problems. It would open up a substantial gap between the out-of-pocket expenses of persons entering SNFs and the expenses of persons entering ICFs, and might, consequently, encourage individuals to exaggerate their impairments in order to qualify for skilled nursing care.

Under our model for the financing of long-term care, both SNF and ICF care benefits would be unlimited in duration. There would be no specific incentive to choose SNF over ICF care; the same cost-sharing formulas would apply to both levels of care. The unlimited stay provision would guarantee the chronically ill and impaired in need of institutional services a high degree of economic security and the peace of mind that comes of that security. On the other hand, the existence of a cost-sharing arrangement would discourage individuals who did not require such intensive care from taking advantage of the benefit.

Another area in which the NHI proposals fall short of meeting the needs of the long-term care population is mental health. Most of the proposals do not provide for unlimited stays in mental hospitals or unlimited outpatient mental health care. Because this type of care may involve very long stays and a large component of custodial care, now provided primarily by the states, most plans restrict coverage to a fairly short period, such as 30 days. There is also apprehension among the drafters of these proposals about the costs of extensive coverage of outpatient psychiatrist and psychologist services. Under our proposal, the states would be required to offer unlimited stays in mental health institutions, including ICF care for the mentally retarded. To guard against overutilization of institutional care, strong financial incentives are built into the system to induce the states to provide alternative services in community and home settings.

Finally, few of the NHI proposals provide benefits for social and supportive services. This is perhaps the most difficult set of services to cover under any traditional health insurance plan. Homemaker, nutrition, transportation, and similar services do not necessarily have to be ordered by physicians, and it is relatively difficult to distinguish those individuals who have a great "need" for these services from those who do not. One NHI proposal that does cover such services calls for the creation of state-regulated, nonprofit, community long-term care centers. Social and homemaker services would be provided through these centers, rather than through the standard health provider market.

The proposal outlined in this chapter is also calculated to encourage maximum use of community and home resources. Increased grants to states and a matching fund mechanism that places the greatest burden on the federal government will enable the states to develop new health and social support services and to expand existing ones. The proposal has the additional advantage of fostering innovative attitudes and responsiveness to local needs. Each state will have the autonomy to design and fund a program of services that is best suited to its resident population.

Conclusion

While the NHI proposals represent a very ambitious effort to reform the federal involvement in the financing of health services for the entire population, they do not come to terms with the needs of the long-term population in an altogether satisfactory way. What is needed is a program recognizing the full implications of chronic illness and disability: the indefinite duration of some conditions and the complicated economic and social ramifications for the individual. The model presented here assures the entire population of financial access to institutional care, at the same time that it discourages inappropriate or excessive reliance on the institutional setting. It acknowledges the value of social and support services, and promotes the development of a wide variety of home and community resources. Finally, the division of financing responsibility under the model grants each level of government primary authority in that area where it can be most effective. So the federal government, in the role of overseeing the institutional component of the program, can enforce uniformity in the costs, quality, and availability of care from state to state. The states, in turn, will have the independence to experiment with different types and combinations of services at the community level.

NOTES

1. U.S., Department of Health, Education, and Welfare, Social Security Administration, Office of Research and Statistics, "Personal Care and Household Needs of the Noninstitutionalized Population," *Social Security Survey of the Disabled: 1966*, Rept. No. 21, DHEW Pubn No. (SSA) 73-11713 (September 1972), p. 7.

2. Ethel Shanas, "Health Status of Older People: Cross-National Implications," *American Journal of Public Health* 64, no. 3 (1974), p. 262.

3. See, for example, John W. Davis and Marilyn J. Gibbin, "An Areawide Examination of Nursing Home Use, Misuse, and Nonuse," *American Journal of Public Health* 61, no. 6 (1971), 1145–55; and Texas Department of Mental Health and Mental Retardation, Final Report of the Study of Placement Needs of State Mental Hospital Patients, NIMH Contract No. (ADM) 42-74-81 (OP), by Danial M. Sheehan and James E. Craft, mimeographed (1974).

4. U.S., Department of Health, Education, and Welfare, Social and Rehabilitation Service, Medical Services Administration, *Medicaid Services by State* (June 1, 1976).

5. U.S., Department of Health, Education, and Welfare, Social and Rehabilitation Service, Office of Information Systems, *Medicaid Statistics, FY 1976* (March 1977), p. 17.

6. U.S., Bureau of the Census, *1970 Census*.

7. U.S., Department of Health, Education, and Welfare, Medical Services Administration, *Medicaid Management Reports: Annual Report FY 1976*, p. 10.

8. U.S., HEW, SRS, *Medicaid Statistics, FY 1976*, p. 6.

9. R.M. Gibson and M.J. Mueller, "National Health Expenditures, FY 1976," *Social Security Bulletin* 40, no. 4 (1977), 3ff.

10. Barry Chiswick, "The Demand for Nursing Home Care," *Journal of Human Resources* 11, no. 3 (1976), 295–316.

11. Total (federal and state) SNF and ICF expenditures are shown in Table 3.1. The $3.0 billion figure is obtained by multiplying the SNF and ICF expenditures by the federal share (56.8 percent) of all Medicaid expenditures. U.S., HEW, MSA, *Medicaid Management Report, FY 1976*, p. 24.

12. Total (federal and state) home health care expenditures are shown in Table 3.1. The $73 million figure is obtained by multiplying the home health care expenditures by the federal share (56.8 percent) of all Medicaid expenditures. U.S., HEW, MSA, *Medicaid Management Report, FY 1976*, p. 24.

4
AN ANALYSIS OF REGULATORY ISSUES AND OPTIONS IN LONG-TERM CARE

Hirsch S. Ruchlin

AN OVERVIEW OF THE LONG-TERM CARE SECTOR

The Long-Term Care Marketplace

The reports recently completed by the Subcommittee on Long-Term Care of the Senate's Special Committee on Aging clearly describe the current state of the long-term care sector.* As noted in the preface to the introductory report:

> . . . public policy has failed to produce satisfactory institutional care—or alternatives—for chronically ill older Americans.
> . . . today's entire population of the elderly, and their offspring, suffer severe emotional damage because of the dread and despair associated with nursing home care in the United States today.
> This policy, or lack thereof, may not be solely responsible for producing such anxiety. Deep-rooted attitudes toward aging and death also play major roles.
> But the actions of Congress and of States, as expressed through the Medicare and Medicaid programs, have in many ways intensified old problems and have created new ones.
> . . . *long-term care for older Americans stands today as the most troubled, and troublesome, component of our entire health care system.*[1]

---

*The subcommittee's report, and the scope of this chapter, focus on one segment of the long-term care marketplace—nursing homes.

Independent of, or possibly as a result of, this lack of sound public policy, additional problems contribute to the industry's troubled state.[2] These problems can be briefly summarized as: unsatisfactory compliance with federal and state codes and standards; inappropriate patient placements; the paucity of suitable alternatives to institutionalization; the limited involvement of the medical and lay communities; the structure of the current reimbursement system, which neither reimburses adequately for the care delivered nor contains incentives for economic efficiency; and the poor implementation of regulatory authority.

Four major consequences can be traced to the cumulative effect of these problems. Owing to facility deficiencies, patient placement in institutions providing a higher level of care than actually required by the patient, and the absence of incentives for efficiency in the current reimbursement system, the price of long-term care services may be excessive for the quality of the product delivered. Facility deficiencies, patient misplacement, and the poor enforcement of existing standards and codes result in a diminution of the quality of the product provided; from both the patient's and the community's viewpoint, the services delivered are often unsatisfactory. The restrained involvement of the medical and lay communities, the presumed absence of concern regarding the effectiveness of the care delivered, the low level of current reimbursement,* and the narrowed reimbursement coverage for noninstitutional care have jointly limited the supply of alternative modes of delivering long-term care services. The meager involvement of the medical and lay communities and the current limited focus of regulatory initiatives result in an environment where concern with the effectiveness of care is minimized. Consequently, patient health status is not as high as it could be if these problems were directly addressed and corrected.

Faced with the industry's persistent ills, the Subcommittee on Long-Term Care has suggested three alternative courses of action.

> The industry could continue to grow as it has in the past, spurred on by sheer need, but marred by scandal, negativism, and murkiness about its fundamental mission.
>
> It could be mandated to transform itself from a predominantly proprietary industry into a nonprofit system, or into one which takes on the attributes of a quasi-public utility.
>
> Or it could—with the informed help of government and the general public—move to overcome present difficulties, to improve standards of performance, and to fit itself successfully into a comprehensive health

---

*The assertion of a low level of reimbursement does not contradict the earlier assertion that the price of long-term care services may be excessive for the quality of the product delivered. While reimbursement rates are often inadequate to ensure a socially acceptable level of care, fraudulent practices and operating inefficiencies may result in a situation of overpayments for the quality of care being provided.

care system in which institutionalization is kept to essential minimums.[3]

The second and third courses of action imply additional regulatory initiatives on the part of the federal and possibly state governments. It is precisely to this course of action that this chapter addresses itself. Prior to embarking on the main analytic sections, a brief historical perspective on long-term care regulation is in order.

Brief History of Long-Term Care Regulation

Institutions providing long-term care services are already subject to substantial government regulation. The bulk of the regulation is by and through state licensure programs, although the enactment of the Medicaid program has introduced federal standards that states are required to adhere to in order to assure continued receipt of federal funds.

Most state licensing statutes date from the early 1950s and were enacted in response to the Social Security Amendments of 1950 that required that every state have a program for the licensing of nursing homes as a condition of participation in the old-age assistance program.[4] Many states also license other facilities providing long-term care; the two principle categories being chronic disease hospitals and personal care domiciliary facilities.

One of the two major amendments to the Social Security Act passed in 1965, and the one having the greatest impact on the long-term care sector, established a federal grant-in-aid program to the states (Title XIX—Medicaid) to help provide medical services for the needy and the medically indigent. The Medicaid program is administered on the national level by the Social and Rehabilitation Service (SRS), Department of Health, Education, and Welfare. A state wishing to participate in the program must submit to SRS a state plan representing its commitment to administer the program in accordance with the provision of Title XIX requirements and related federal regulations and policies. SRS is responsible for approving state plans and for providing guidance and assistance to the state agencies responsible for administering the Medicaid program. (As of June 1977, the newly established Health Care Financing Administration has replaced SRS as the federal agency with responsibility for the Medicaid program.) Facilities providing skilled nursing care were immediately included in the Medicaid program; facilities providing intermediate care (a less intensive level of care) became eligible for incorporation into the program in 1971.[5] Two essential elements of the Medicaid program are that the federal role is essentially limited to interaction with the states rather than with the providers and/or recipients of care, and that the establishment and maintenance of quality of care standards is a state rather than a federal responsibility.[6]

Having briefly noted some of the major problems characteristic of the long-term care sector, and the legislative basis for government regulation, we now focus attention on the regulatory process and the effectiveness of regulatory efforts in other sectors of the economy.

REGULATION: INTRODUCTION

One of the most **significant** phenomena in the evolution of U.S. industry in the last one hundred years has been the growth of public regulation of economic life. The conventional justification for regulation is the improvement of the performance of the economy, in both practical and welfare terms. However, the mere existence of regulatory authority and mechanisms does not, by itself, necessarily guarantee the desired industry performance. The material presented in this section focuses on analyses of existing regulatory mechanisms in an attempt to determine both whether major national regulatory efforts have been successful, and possible explanations for the reported effectiveness of economic regulation.

Regulatory Experiences in Other Sectors of the Economy

There seems to be fairly wide agreement among students of industrial organization that public (utility) regulation has either had no effect on industry performance or has imposed considerable costs on company operations without providing compensating benefits to the public.[7] It is also alleged that regulation removes any stimulus for cost-cutting innovations and often prevents new firms with innovative products or processes from entering the regulated industry.[8] One indication of the failure of regulation efforts is provided by recent estimates of the economic waste attributable to the regulation of the transportation and communications industry that place the loss in the range of $16 to $24 billion.[9]

It is worth noting that the regulatory mechanisms that have been scrutinized and critiqued in the literature have been directed at basic economic phenomena such as prices, profits, and entry. Only recently has attention been directed to the question of what happens to the quality attributes of a product when conventional regulation is imposed.[10] Clear empirical answers to this question are not yet available.

Theories of Regulation

Why have the traditional attempts at industry regulation failed? A review of the theories of regulation provides some insights into this phenomenon. Whereas the simplistic view of regulation assumes that the goal is to protect the public interest, students of regulation view the process as an arena where various "actors" attempt to maximize their self-interest. For analytic purposes it is convenient to group the theories into two categories: dominant interest group theories and participatory interest group theories.

Proponents of dominant interest group theories agree that initially or ultimately, one group or a coalition dominates the regulatory process and subverts it to its desires. Bernstein and Jaffe assert that the regulators ultimately recognize that their survival is dependent on their willingness to accept and champion the viewpoint of the regulated.[11] Thus, the regulated "capture" the regulators and dominate the regulatory process. Stigler asserts that the industry (the regulated) desire regulation for the benefits they expect it to bestow upon them and demand it, as it is in their best economic self-interest.[12] Posner accepts Stigler's hypothesis that regulation is demanded by industry, but expands the theory of economic regulation by recognizing a quid pro quo in the process of granting regulation.[13] This quid pro quo, called "taxation by regulation," entails the continued provision of unprofitable services in some markets out of profits reaped from providing services in other markets. In effect, the regulated and the regulator jointly dominate the regulatory process at the expense of the public. Baldwin and Wilson disagree with the "capture" and "self-interest" theories and assert that the process is ultimately affected, if not controlled, by the regulatory bureaucracy (the regulators).[14] Wilson asserts that:

> . . . the term 'capture' reflects a simplistic view of the politics of regulation. Though there have been very few good studies of agency politics, what probably happens is this: An agency is established, sometimes with industry support and sometimes over industry objections, and then gradually creates a regulatory climate that acquires a life of its own. Certain firms will be helped by some of the specific regulatory decisions making up this climate, others will be hurt. But the industry as a whole will adjust to the climate and decide that the costs of shifting from the known hazards of regulation to the unknown ones of competition are too great; it thus will come to defend the system. The agencies themselves will become preoccupied with the details of regulation and the minutiae of cases in whatever forms they first inherit them, trying by the slow manipulation of detail to achieve various particular effects that happen to commend themselves from time to time to various regulatory agency members.
>
> . . . the agencies are not so much industry-oriented or consumer-oriented as *regulation-oriented*. They are in the regulation business, and regulate they will, with or without a rationale. If the agencies have been 'captured' by anybody, it is probably by their staffs who have mastered the arcane details of rate setting and license granting.[15]

Without necessarily disputing the emergence of a dominant interest group, some social theorists believe that the nature of regulation cannot really be understood unless it is viewed as a process.[16] These theories can be characterized as focusing on participatory rather than dominant interest groups.

Bernstein conceives of the process in terms of a "life cycle." The first period—gestation—is marked by slowly mounting public pressure for action with regard to a specific social problem. Public pressure continues to mount leading to the creation of an agency of regulation. However, the desire for regulation and the drive to establish a regulatory entity takes precedence over attempts to refine regulatory goals and policies. Thus, a short-run rather than long-run perspective guides the exercise of regulatory power from its inception. Three distinct attributes characterize the second phase—youth. The regulatory agency, as it begins its administrative career, exhibits an aggressive, crusading spirit in dealing with regulatory problems. However, the animosities generated during the period of gestation do not subside, and the regulators are reminded of the strength of the regulated groups at every possible opportunity. Concomitantly, public attention to the regulated industry begins to fade and consequently, public support of regulatory initiatives declines. The third phase—maturity—is marked by the process of agency devitalization. The regulatory agency adjusts to the conflict atmosphere and functions less as a police officer and more as a manager. Public passivity gives way to apathy and the "capture" process (Bernstein's hypothesis) begins. In the fourth phase—old age—the agency, finding itself abandoned by the public, opts for safety in policy decisions. Public apathy encourages budgetary retrenchment on the part of the legislature. Debility and senescence are now the prevalent characteristics of the regulatory agency.

Implications for the Long-Term Care Sector

While the necessity of a government initiative to guarantee the health and safety of a population cohort is widely recognized, it is clear that the *traditional* regulatory model is not a promising route. The regulatory agency eventually ceases to function in the public interest, and economic waste may become the major byproduct of regulation. However, these findings focus on *economic* regulation and do not necessarily imply that new regulatory approaches focused on noneconomic issues are necessarily doomed to fail.

In attempting to design new regulatory initiatives, it is wise to consider two obsrvations offered by former commissioners of regulatory agencies. The conclusions they have drawn from their experience are very much in line with the formulations of the theoriests cited earlier: all emphasize the significant role played by economic self-interest in the regulation process. Lee Loevinger, former Commissioner of the Federal Communications Commission, observes that

> The regulatory function must accommodate to the fact that economic man is motivated by self-interest, that he seeks his own profit and that he is entitled to do so. These motives must be harnessed to the achievement of the objectives sought.[17]

Robert Ball, former Commissioner of the Social Security Administration, echoes these sentiments. He notes that.

> . . . realistically we should not be choosing between the market, with its emphasis on incentives, and regulation, with its emphasis on directions and sanctions. I would guess that regulation that attempts to accomplish an objective by fiat, swimming upstream against a powerful current of opposing incentives, has little chance of success. But regulation that is consistent with or creates motivation that moves in the desired direction may be a different matter. Perhaps the task in the immediate future will be to strengthen incentives, competition, and choices and yet introduce direct regulation related to a relatively small number of major strategic points, seeking to avoid the rigidities that could develop in regulating the details of such a highly complicated system as health care delivery.[18]

A number of regulatory efforts focused on major strategic points have already been directed at the acute care health system. We review these initiatives in the next section in order to determine whether the desired goals were achieved, and whether any or all of these regulatory initiatives are appropriate for the long-term care setting.

REGULATION IN THE ACUTE HEALTH CARE SECTOR

Introduction

The contemporary hospital has been subject to extensive regulatory programs from all levels and branches of government for many years. However, the regulatory climate has recently changed from one that was viewed as relatively innocuous to one that seeks to clearly circumscribe institutional behavior and performance. The turning point in the regulatory environment can be traced to the unexpected and unwelcome hospital cost spiral that resulted from the passage of the Medicare/Medicaid legislation.

The breadth of regulatory control that has existed in the acute health care sector is indicated by the findings of an unpublished study conducted by the American Hospital Association in 1968, which identified 68 different hospital programs or facilities affected by direct government controls. The areas of control, and the number of regulatory programs were: physical plant and equipment—18, reporting—13, permit to operate—12, personnel—12, working conditions—9, and miscellaneous—4.[19] Nongovernment agencies such as the Joint Commission on Accreditation of Hospitals, the American Medical Association, and the National League for Nursing further constrain hospital activities by establishing standards in their respective areas of jurisdiction.

Recent efforts to control hospital activities have been directed at changing the rate setting process to institute cost controls, controlling capital expenditures, and reviewing professional performance. These regulatory thrusts merit review as they seek to directly modify institutional performance, and exist or can be implemented in the long-term care sector.

Cost Controls

Various cost control programs have been initiated on a national or state basis in an attempt to limit hospital cost increases. On the federal level, the most dramatic effort of recent times was the Economic Stabilization Program (ESP), introduced in August 1971 and terminated in April 1974. During this period, a wage and price freeze, and later, wage and price controls, were imposed on hospitals. Comparisons of hospital cost increases in the ESP and pre-ESP periods appear to indicate that the hospital cost spiral was being harnessed. However, an in-depth exploration of the process by which this cost containment was achieved fails to identify the Economic Stabilization Program as the crucial element.

A study undertaken by Stuart Altman and Joseph Eichenholz examined increases in hospital expenditures during the period 1963–74. Although this analysis was completed prior to the termination of ESP, it indicates substantial declines in expenses for each adjusted patient day, expenses for each adjusted admission, intensity of services for each patient day, and to a limited extent in intensity of services per admission during the ESP periods as compared to the pre-ESP periods.[20] As a result of these findings the authors imply that the Economic Stabilization Program was a success. One other interpretation of these findings is possible, however. The reduction in the rate of cost increases might be attributed to the reduction—also recorded by the authors—in the rate of increase in input intensity, or intensity of services. Input intensity is clearly the quantity dimension in the quality of care phenomenon, the other dimension being a pure quality increase in a constant input level. If cost controls affect the quality of care provided, and if the existent quality of care is deemed to be inadequate, then the victory achieved may, from a broadened perspective, prove to be quite hollow.

Research conducted by Paul Ginsburg on hospital cost trends over the period 1969–73 appears to support the findings of Altman and Eichenholz. Ginzburg reports a decline in the rate of increase of both revenue for each adjusted patient day, and cost for each adjusted patient day.[21] However, when the time series data are subjected to econometric analysis, the reported declines in input intensity, costs, and prices were small and generally not significant. Ginzburg further notes that the only important reduction in cost appeared to result from a decline in mean stay, but he questions whether this reduction occurred as a result of ESP.[22]

The second broad attempt to control costs on a national level is being implemented through the Medicare reimbursement process. Under the authority granted in Section 223 of P.L. 92-603, the Secretary of Health, Education, and Welfare has set limits on hospital reimbursement for routine costs in such areas as maintenance, laundry and linen, housekeeping, dietary, medical records, central services, pharmacy, and administration. No published studies have appeared to date assessing the effectiveness of this attempt at mitigating the hospital cost spiral.

The major state effort at cost containment via the Medicaid rate setting process is the formula approach to prospective reimbursement adopted by New York State in 1969. Under the New York State formula, hospitals are grouped by type, size, ownership, and geographic location and the routine costs of each hospital are allowed only up to 110 percent of the group mean. Historical costs are "trended forward" to permit the establishment of a prospective rate.

A recent evaluation of the New York experience conducted by Berry indicates that as a result of the formula-prospective approach, price and cost increases have been moderated, and the rate of increase of inputs has been particularly slowed.[23] Recognizing the existence of the national ESP effort that was operative during the 1971–74 period, Berry reported that the cost increases occurring in New York were significantly less than national and select regional cost increases during this period. Thus, he concludes that the local reimbursement changes had the desired effect. It is noteworthy that the effect of the New York State approach was severe enough to result in some hospital deficits during the study period (1970–74).[24] The possible effect of reduced rates of input intensity on quality of care has already been noted; the probable effect of the incurred deficits is in the same direction, namely, a reduction in the overall quality of care provided.*

---

*Increased productivity could *temporarily* offset the postulated adverse effect of these two developments on the quality of care rendered. However, if constant pressure is applied to lower costs, the quality of care will ultimately be reduced.

Prospective reimbursement systems have also been established in 21 other states, either under the auspices of the state health department, or the local Blue Cross plan, or both.[25] A number of the programs have been established on a permanent basis; others are experimental and subject to review after a number of years of experience. A recent survey of the effects of these systems on hospital costs reported that no conclusive quantitative evidence existed to indicate that rate review systems (which include the utilization of the prospective reimbursement approach) contain costs.[26] Some subjective evaluations indicate that limited success has been achieved in a number of instances in effecting some cost containment. Similar conclusions emerge from the ten "case studies" of prospective reimbursement of hospitals (excluding New York) conducted by Katherine Bauer, Arva Clark, and Arthur D. Little, Inc.[27]

Regulation of Capital Expenditures

Two major programs currently exist for regulating the construction, expansion, or modification of health care facilities and for the purchase of capital equipment. They are the various state certificate-of-need statutes establishing state designated agencies with the above-noted regulatory powers, and the 1122 Review Program created by Section 221 of P.L. 92-603, which requires the approval by a state-designated agency of capital expenditures exceeding $100,000 in order for such expenditures to be considered as reimbursable under the Medicare program. Both of these functions—the administration of a state certificate-of-need program and the 1122 review—have been delegated to the designated Health Systems Agencies that have been established in conformance with Section 1523 of P.L. 93-641, the National Health Planning and Resources Development Act of 1974.

The rationale for attempting to regulate capital expenditures is the perceived excess utilization of capital inputs in the health care industry and the effect this excess utilization has on health care costs. Excess utilization exists in the sense of duplication of expensive facilities and equipment. Capital expenditures commit the institution to a series of operating expenses—labor and supplies—and within the health field, supply often creates its own demand. That is, the existence of a capital item—a bed or equipment—is usually enough to guarantee its utilization, as physicians can be encouraged to validate the wisdom of the capital expenditure decision.

As of 1975, twenty-nine states and the District of Columbia had enacted certificate-of-need legislation,[28] and 39 states had also implemented 1122 review programs.[29] A preliminary evaluation of these programs in the aggregate has indicated a lack of clear and refined criteria that are used in assessing need and a lack of an adequate budget to support such regulatory tasks.[30] These problems notwithstanding, providers of care, consumer groups, and regulatory agency representatives agreed that these programs had made a positive contribution to the regulatory environment and had achieved some success in reducing unnecessary construction and duplication of facilities.[31]

The apparent support by providers of care of capital expenditure regulation may initially appear puzzling, in light of their traditional reluctance to accept government control. It is not at all puzzling if one accepts the hypothesis advanced by Havighurst that certificate-of-need agencies will have no incentive to do more than bring about conditions roughly equivalent to those that a hospital cartel would maintain if it could.[32] The support of certificate-of-need legislation by state hospital associations tends to lend face validity to Havighurst's hypothesis.[33]

Some recent empirical evidence presented by Salkever and Bice lends some indirect support to the cartel hypothesis and also casts doubt on the success of capital expenditure regulation. Utilizing data for the period 1968–72, they estimated the impact of state certificate-of-need programs on three different measures of capital investment: change in plant assets, change in bed supply, and change in assets for each bed. Their econometric analysis implies that the effect of a certificate-of-need program over the entire four-year period was to reduce growth in beds by 3.5 to 9.0 percent and to increase assets for each bed by 10 to 19.7 percent.[34] The authors conclude that certificate-of-need programs clearly have not reduced total hospital investment. Rather they have skewed the capital expansion process and appear to favor the expansion plans of those providers who are already in the industry.

Licensure, Certification, and Accreditation

Licensure, certification, and accreditation are all aimed at the basic objective of establishing minimal standards of institutional performance. The presumed market deficiency to which these regulatory programs are directed is the problem of ensuring an adequate level of quality of care. Licensure has the specific objective of controlling the opening of new facilities and of enforcing minimal standards among operating facilities. Accreditation, which is primarily a voluntary program operated by the Joint Commission on Accreditation of Hospitals (JCAH), has the additional objective of encouraging providers to maintain standards at a level that is somewhat higher than minimal licensing criteria. Certification has as its objective the entitlement to participate in a program such as Medicare or

Medicaid, and is obtained by a process which resembles, or is identical with, accreditation.*

Analyses of both licensure and certification/accreditation programs indicate a number of shortcomings. Facility inspections, a prerequisite for licensing and relicensing, focus largely on physical plant, safety, and structural elements of hospitals. Rarely are standards set or included in the inspection process for gauging adequate levels of medical care. Where such standards exist there is a general laxity in enforcement.[35] Furthermore, low budget appropriations in state regulatory agencies cause staffing deficiencies and sporadic enforcement, and low pay scales dissuade highly qualified persons from becoming employed as inspectors.[36]

JCAH accreditation is voluntary. About 2,200 hospitals, nearly one-third of the total in the United States, fail to meet JCAH standards but still continue to render medical and surgical care.[37] JCAH standards themselves are questioned and attacked for their failure to examine the quality of care "output" of hospitals. One study, conducted by Roemer, Moustafa, and Hopkins, found that very little difference in terms of quality exists between the care provided by JCAH-accredited hospitals and that provided by nonaccredited hospitals.[38]

Recent court settlements of malpractice suits have emphasized the failure of existing mechanisms to prevent gross hospital negligence and incompetence, and have prodded the JCAH to establish some well-defined quality control procedures as requirements for accreditation.[39] However, no empirical evidence is available to indicate the effectiveness of this recent shift in JCAH emphasis.

Peer Review

Peer review entails the monitoring of professional performance by one's peers. The intent of peer review is to preserve and improve quality standards, and secondarily, to see that medical services are not over-utilized. Two peer review mechanisms are relevant for the current analysis: they are utilization review and medical audit. Both of these functions now fall within the domain of the Professional Standards Review Organizations (PSROs) mandated in Section 249F of P.L. 92-603.

---

*Accreditation by the Joint Commission on Accreditation of Hospitals (JCAH) and certification of hospitals as providers for the purpose of reimbursement for services rendered to Medicare beneficiaries are practically synonymous, as the Secretary of Health, Education, and Welfare, in general, may not set certification requirements that are higher than JCAH standards. (Section 1861 (e) (5) of the Social Security Act of 1965). JCAH standards thus become the conditions for participation by hospitals in the Medicare program.

There appears to be widespread recognition of the fact that the traditional peer review mechanisms have generally failed to change professional behavior. One explanation for this failure is the lack of commitment on the part of reviewers to expose their errant colleagues or to offer a critical assessment.[40] While it is still too early to evaluate the effectiveness of PSROs, it is significant that many of the PSROs that have been established are operated or dominated by representatives of local medical societies. Medical societies have traditionally been reluctant to engage in any effective self-policing activities.[41] It is quite likely that any standards set by PSROs will be at the least common denominator and overlooked whenever possible.

Implications for Long-Term Care Regulation

A number of students of the U.S. health scene have advocated the adoption of a public utility model for regulating hospitals and nursing homes.[42] Many of the regulatory levers of the public utility approach—rate and capital investment regulation—already exist in the health field, and others usually not associated with public utility regulation—accreditation/certification and peer review—have also been implemented. With the possible exception of rate regulation, all these regulatory mechanisms have failed to elicit the desired industry behavior.

The one regulatory approach that appears to offer some promise of success is rate setting. There is evidence to suggest, however, that its effectiveness has been at the expense of quality of care. One possible means of remedying this problem would be to create certain procedural linkages that would tie the concern for quality of care with the rate-setting function. Such linkages would be necessary to ensure that cost control brings about a reduction in operating inefficiencies, rather than in the quality of care.

The usefulness of this suggested approach extends also to long-term care; we return to it in the last section of the chapter after our review of the existing regulatory mechanisms in the long-term care sector.

REGULATION IN THE LONG-TERM HEALTH CARE SECTOR

Federal/State Regulatory Powers

The long-term care sector of the health industry is already subject to significant regulatory statutes emanating from federal and state governments. In order to be eligible to participate in, and receive reimbursement for, skilled nursing care rendered through the Medicare and/or Medicaid programs, a facility must meet certain "conditions for participation" or regulatory guidelines specified jointly by the Social Security Administration (SSA) and the Social and Rehabilitation Service (SRS). These requirements are detailed in Code of Federal Regulations, Title 20, Chapter II, Part 405, Subpart K. From the vantage point of SSA, these conditions must be met for a facility to be certified for participation in the Medicare program. From the vantage point of SRS these conditions are guidelines that should be embodied in individual state Medicaid plans. However, SRS must approve these plans for states to qualify for and receive federal grant-in-aid funds. Most of the state plans embody, to a greater or lesser extent, the SRS guidelines as state standards. (As of June 1977, the Health Care Financing Administration has assumed these responsibilities previously held by SSA and SRS.) As of June 1975, conditions and standards have been specified for 18 major areas. These areas and their primary focus are detailed in Table 4.1.

TABLE 4.1

Specific Areas Specified in Conditions of Participation for Skilled Nursing Facilities

Section	Area	Focus
405.1120	Compliance with federal, state, and local laws	Licensure; registration of personnel; health and safety requirements.
405.1121	Governing Body and Management	Disclosure of ownership; staffing patterns; bylaws; medical review; administrator; institutional planning; personnel policies; use of outside resources; notification of change in patient's status; patient's rights; patient-care policies.
405.1122	Medical Direction	Retainment of a full- or part-time medical director; coordination of medical care.
405.1123	Physician Services	Physicians' orders; patient supervision; availability of physician for emergency care.
405.1124	Nursing Services	Responsibilities of director of nursing; designation and function of charge nurse; nursing coverage; development of patient-care plan; rehabilitative nursing care; supervision of patient nutrition; administration of of drugs; drug orders; storage of drugs and biologicals.

Section	Area	Focus
405.1125	Dietetic Services	Staffing; nutritional adequacy; therapeutic diets; frequency of meals; food preparation and service; sanitary conditions.
405.1126	Specialized Rehabilitation Services	Staffing; plan of care; documentation of services.
405.1127	Pharmaceutical Services	Supervision and services; control and accountability; labeling of drugs; policies and procedures.
405.1128	Laboratory and Radiologic Services	Provision for services; blood products and blood handling.
405.1129	Dental Services	Dental health policies; arrangements for outside services.
405.1130	Social Services	Functions; staffing; records.
405.1131	Patient Activities	Responsibility; provision of program.
405.1132	Medical Records	Staffing; record content; physician documentation.
405.1133	Transfer Agreement	Patient transfer.
405.1134	Physical Environment	Life safety; emergency power; facilities for physically handicapped; nursing unit; patient rooms and toilet facilities; facilities for special care; dining and patient activities rooms; kitchen and dietetic service; maintenance of equipment, buildings, and grounds; other environmental factors.
405.1135	Infection Control	Committee composition and function; aseptic and isolation techniques; housekeeping; linen; pest control.
405.1136	Disaster Preparedness	Disaster plan; staff training and drills.
405.1137	Utilization Review	Activity plan; committee composition; medical care evaluation studies; review of extended stay cases; discharge planning.

Source: U.S. Department of Health, Education, and Welfare. *Interpretive Guidelines and Survey Procedures for the Application of the Conditions of Participation for Skilled Nursing Facilities*. Mimeographed, June 17, 1975.

In addition to setting standards (as absolute requirements or guidelines to be followed), the federal government formulates interpretive guidelines intended to indicate to the state survey agencies and Medicaid agencies the intent of the promulgated standard and a suggested survey procedure to ascertain compliance.

The federal conditions of participation have undergone some basic changes since their initial promulgation at the inception of the Medicare/ Medicaid programs. The major changes that are likely to have a direct impact on quality of care have been in the areas of medical direction (Section 405.1122) and patient's right (Section 405.1121(k)). Other sections have been modified or expanded to elucidate the federal intent but do not constitute a significant advancement or retraction of the scope of regulatory authority.

SRS has also issued recommended basic standards for inclusion in state Medicaid plans as a basis for certifying facilities rendering intermediate nursing care as eligible to participate in the Medical Assistance Program (Medicaid). Because intermediate-care facilities are expected to provide a less intensive level of care, the specific standards promulgated for their observance are usually less stringent.

State regulatory authority stems from individual state public health statutes and codes and from the state's authorized role as the executor and interpretor of SRS guidelines. State health commissioners have the authority to issue, deny, and renew an operating license, and inspect facilities to determine conformance with code and standard requirements. In addition, state public health codes grant the commissioner power to promulgate such rules and regulations deemed necessary for the protection of life, health, and welfare of institutionalized persons and for the successful implementation of health and welfare laws.*

It appears that existing standards or conditions of participation cover a wide spectrum of areas that circumscribes institutional behavior. State authorities are empowered to propose and implement any rules, regulations, and standards deemed necessary. Authority exists at the state level to ensure adherence to these regulations by threatening to revoke a license or, in some states, through the imposition of penalties.† Thus, adequate

---

*Thirty-nine states responded to a mail inquiry addressed to each state's health commissioner requesting copies of state codes detailing their regulatory powers in the long-term care field. In every case authority existed to license facilities. In all but three instances, authoriy existed to revoke or suspend a license, adopt and enforce standards, and inspect faciliies. The three exceptions encountered are probably the result of the submission of incomplete information rather than the absence of authority.

†Of the 39 state health commissioners responding to the inquiry on regulatory authority, 21 appear to have the authority to invoke penalties or fines as a means of ensuring conformance with the enacted regulations. The other 18 commissioners may also have such authority but failed to submit any reference to it.

regulatory authority appears to exist currently and has existed since the implementation of the Medicare/Medicaid programs. Unfortunately, existence alone does not ensure implementation, for there is a wide gap between what has been legislated and what prevails in the real world.

The Failure of Existing Regulatory Efforts

Despite the clear requirement that facilities must comply with the conditions of participation/standards to be eligible for participation in the Medicare/Medicaid programs, facilities have been receiving federal and state reimbursement payments when it has been documented that the necessary compliance has not been attained. HEW audit studies have uncovered such situations in Indiana, Kentucky, Massachusetts, and Rhode Island.[43] The extent of the regulatory failure is clearly stated in the Indiana audit report.

> Medicaid criteria do not permit entering into more than two successive 6-month agreements with facilities that are cited for deficiencies. Our examination disclosed that the State Agency issued as many as three successive agreements over periods that, in the aggregate, ranged from 22 to 32 months. . . . Our review also disclosed that contrary to program criteria, second agreements were executed with nursing homes where the same deficiencies continued for two or more consecutive inspections. In 17 of the 24 nursing homes, the same 69 deficiencies were noted by the SBH [State Board of Health] during four successive inspections. The SBH reports, however, did not recommend withholding certifications. Consequently, the State Agency continued to issue certification agreements to these homes without any documented evidence that the nursing homes had made substantial effort and progress in correcting these deficiencies. The deficiences were in 11 of the 18 Conditions of Participation which are part of the Medicaid criteria designed to insure that nursing homes are capable of providing skilled nursing care and services.[44]

Widespread deficiencies with respect to compliance with Life Safety Code requirements are a commonplace phenomenon in the long-term care field and were attributed, in the past, to the fact that many nursing homes were constructed in periods when such conformance was not required. The fact remains, however, that these conditions continue to exist. A recent audit conducted in the state of New Hampshire noted that 71 nursing home facilities did not meet Life Safety Code requirements.[45] The study of Rhode Island facilities noted that many intermediate-care facilities do not meet numerous fire safety requirements; similar findings were reported for skilled nursing facilities located in Idaho.[46]

The basic requirement that patients receive periodic medical examinations is another example of a regulatory requirement that is not met. An examination of a sample of Medicaid records in the state of Minnesota indicated that 78 percent of the patients requiring skilled nursing care had not been seen by their physicians at regular 30 day intervals, as required by federal regulations.[47] Similar failures to meet the required standard were noted in Maine, Kentucky, Idaho, Illinois, and Oregon.[48] The net result of the inadequate attention given to patients by physicians is poor medical care: physicians fail to evaluate patients, fail to monitor therapy, and sometimes fail to diagnose new ailments that occur subsequent to a patient's entry into a nursing home. Furthermore, the absence of the physician also has a detrimental effect on the quality of nursing care by imposing functions on the nursing staff that they are inadequately prepared to fulfill.[49]

The failure of utilization review to guarantee appropriate placement is a further regulatory deficiency. Patients may be placed in a facility providing a higher level of care than they require, or in a facility that is not equipped to provide the care needed. In the first instance, public funds are being wasted as the reimbursement payments for this patient are unnecessarily high, and in the second instance, inadequate care is being rendered. The HEW audit reports conducted in Georgia, Illinois, Indiana, Maryland, Minnesota, Oregon, Rhode Island, Utah, Virginia, and West Virginia indicate the widespread nature of the violation of this condition of participation/standard.[50]

Noncompliance with the conditions of participation/standards promulgated in the dietary, pharmacy, and housekeeping areas have also been reported for a number of states in both the Subcommittee on Long-Term Care reports[51] and in individual HEW audit studies.[52] Noncompliance with requirements for physical therapy services was reported in the Indiana audit report and the New York State Moreland Act Commission study.[53]

Widespread violations of patient personal and property rights have also been reported.[54] These violations include abuse and poor treatment of patients, deliberate physical injury, misappropriation and theft of personal funds, unauthorized or improper use of restraints, reprisals against those who complain, and assaults on human dignity. Although the elaboration of patients' rights in the conditions of participation did not occur until the October 1975 revisions, activities that threaten the health and safety of patients have always been considered violations of the promulgated standards and codes.

The full extent of the failure of existing regulation is indicated by the assertion of the Subcommittee on Long-Term Care that over 50 percent of U.S. nursing homes have *serious* and *life-threatening*, as opposed to technical, violations.[55] Subcommittee members further asserted that the HEW standards are minimal rather than maximum ones.[56]

Factors Limiting the Effectiveness of Existing Regulatory Efforts

Many explanations have been offered for the persistent failure of federal and state regulatory efforts to improve the level of nursing home care. These explanations can be grouped under two broad headings: factors asociated with the nature of the regulatory process and structural barriers to the effective implementation of regulatory powers.

The effectiveness of the current regulatory process rests on the ability to carry out meaningful inspections, for it is primarily through the inspection process that "feedback" data are obtained on the performance of the industry. Such data can then be used to evaluate compliance with the regulatory requirements and to develop additional approaches to improving industry behavior. Internal and external factors tend to negate the effectiveness of the inspection process. These factors can be summarized as inadequate financing, an inadequate knowledge base, bureaucratic apathy, problems associated with the concerns and functioning of the legal process, and the exertion of political influence by the regulated; and they affect the inspection process in both direct and indirect ways.

The effectiveness of any inspection process is greatly limited by the manpower pool that is available to conduct the inspections. Limiting the manpower pool automatically constrains the nature of the inspection process in that inspections are conducted less frequently, and the scope of the inspection is undoubtedly narrowed. Virtually every state agency entrusted with inspection responsibilities is understaffed. The Subcommittee on Long-Term Care reported that in 1971 there were two people assigned to visit 136 nursing homes in Utah.[57] The state of New Jersey currently employs 28 inspectors to oversee the performance of approximately 400 facilities. New York has dramatically strengthened its inspection process during 1975 as a result of the recent public attention directed at nursing home abuses in the state. The state currently employs a professional staff of 200 inspectors to oversee a long-term care sector that includes approximately 1,500 providers (not all of whom are nursing homes). Health Department officials feel that they would need to hire an additional 548 professionals at an added cost of 9 million dollars a year to achieve adequate staffing for a thorough and effective inspection process.[58]

An inadequate knowledge base exists to support an effective inspection process. The inspection process prevailing in most states is concentrated on evaluating the physical plant and the written procedures and internal documents that detail procedures for complying with promulgated standards. Very little attention is given to the quality of patient care and the type of environment or quality of life prevailing in the facility. Two explanations can be offered for this narrowed focus. First, the existing standards barely focus on such issues; and second, inadequate measures exist for determining quality of patient care and quality of life. Consequently, one cannot devise inspection protocols that seek to measure or evaluate these intangible, but crucial, elements.

Some HEW-sponsored research has recently been completed that seeks to expand the focus of inspections to include detailed patient assessment.[59] Five major categories are delineated as the basis for patient assessment: identifying and sociodemographic items, functioning status items, impairment items, medical status and risk factors, and the existence of certain medically defined conditions. The Office of Nursing Home Affairs (DHEW) recently utilized this patient classification model as part of an attempt to ascertain patients' needs for care associated with their pathophysiologic and psychosocial conditions.[60] Through a stratified random sampling process, 283,915 patients in skilled nursing facilities were selected as the sample for the study. In order to implement the survey, a special team of inspectors was recruited and given intensive training for a period of one to three days. The actual data-collection process entailed a commitment by the inspection team of 8–16 hours for each facility. While this approach, which admittedly is quite costly, entailed a significant and pioneering advance in reorienting the inspection process toward the patient and the patient's needs rather than the facility, it is still inadequate as a model for assessing patient needs. In order to assess patient care needs from a comprehensive perspective, attention still must be paid to three major areas that should complement the medical/nursing focus of the patient classification model. These areas are the existing social factors that prompt institutionalization, the need for environmental support, and the patient's own inner strengths and weaknesses. Without these three areas, utilization review will be incomplete, for it will not be possible to correctly assess either the need for institutionalization or the degree of care and supervision required.

To date, no state appears to be adopting the focus proposed in the patient assessment document. Most states still orient their inspections to an assessment of the physical plant and a review of written protocols. In effect, the states are following the traditional Joint Commission on Accreditation of Hospitals approach by assuming that compliance with established physical plant and protocol requirements ensures that facilities have the *capability* of rendering good care, whether or not acceptable and humane care is, in fact, delivered. However, in many states, clear guidelines do not exist to ensure that even such a narrowly focused inspection can be properly implemented. The Moreland Act Commission investigating nursing home care in New York noted that the health department failed to clearly define and grade deficiencies in terms of severity, and develop an enforcement policy with respect to repeatedly found deficiencies.[61] An HEW audit of Massachusetts' certification program for skilled nursing facilities noted a similar problem. It concluded that no clear understanding existed of what constitutes a deficiency in health and safety indicators. The audit report suggested that a state agency should establish criteria that would permit an evaluation of whether unmet items are serious enough to constitute a deficiency in federal requirements.[62]

While it is a tedious and time-consuming process to develop specific guidelines for the inspection process and to reorient the inspection procedure to patient care—quality-of-life elements, the slow progress made to date is traceable, in part, to the relatively low priority and limited funding given to such knowledge generation.

Bureaucratic apathy further affects the effectiveness of the inspection process. The Senate Subcommittee on Long-Term Care noted that in many states inspections are cursory or pro forma. When inspectors did submit negative reports and recommended license revocation or other disciplinary action, little or no follow-up action was instituted.[63] Unwillingness to either invoke fines, revoke licenses, or institute other measures to assure compliance was reported in studies of the nursing home industry in Minnesota, Maryland, Illinois, Indiana, Massachusetts, Rhode Island, New York, and New Jersey.[64] Significantly, where strict measures were taken, such as the imposition of fines or the refusal to relicense homes, the desired results were achieved.[65] The inadequate financing of the regulatory process undoubtedly limits a state agency's ability to follow up on recommendations for disciplinary action and helps to create an atmosphere of resignation and apathy among the state's inspectors.

The circuitous nature of the legal process and the apparent championing of owner's property rights over patient's rights to quality care, further hamper the effectiveness of the regulatory process and indirectly contribute to the prevalence of bureaucratic apathy among inspectors and regulators.[66] Most states cannot act against a substandard facility except through lengthy and costly formal procedures for license revocation or closing.[67] Inadequate funding often precludes such a course of action. The courts, at least in some states, appear to be placing the burden of proof in such cases upon the state, and the previously noted lack of clarity concerning the standards applied during the inspection process often weakens the state's claims vis-a-vis the property rights claim of operators.[68] Even when the operator/owner of a facility has been convicted of a felony, and the state actively attempts to remove an operating license, legal obstacles and appeals can prevent or delay the facility's closing.

The exertion of political influence on the part of the regulated to negate regulatory directives further hampers the functioning of the regulatory agency and reinforces the climate of bureaucratic apathy. A witness appearing before the Subcommittee on Long-Term Care reported that political pressure exerted by an elected official on the Department of Public Health resulted in the relicensure of a nursing home facility in Illinois in spite of consistent inspection reports spanning a period of four years in which major violations were noted and recommendations for closing the facility were made.[69] An Ohio State Senator apparently admitted that legislative influence was being purchased in his state by the nursing home industry.[70] The reputed connections between an indicted nursing home operator in New York State and the state governor's office has been one explanation for the state's passivity in policing the activities of this individual and his nursing home "empire."[71]

Political influence is often exerted in more subtle manners. Recent legislative initiatives in New York have radically changed the overall regulatory environment. Strong fines are being imposed and legislation has been enacted permitting class-action suits against nursing homes. As a result of these initiatives, the association of proprietary nursing homes has asserted that its members cannot operate under these conditions, and many owners want to sell their facilities to nonprofit organizations.[72] State health department officials believe that this position does not constitute an idle threat. However, nonprofit organizations have been reluctant to take over proprietary nursing homes unless they are guaranteed high reimbursement levels.[73] Thus, the health department is now in an awkward position. Unable to guarantee high reimbursement rates, it finds that there is no practical alternative to owners of proprietary facilities that are unwilling to improve the level of care provided in their facilities. This realization also pervades the ranks of the state's inspectors.

The cumulative weight of the evidence presented on the reasons for the ineffectiveness of the regulatory environment in the long-term care sector strongly implies that long-term care regulation has clearly passed through the first three phases of the Bernstein regulatory "life-cycle" schema and is on the verge of, or within, phase four—debility and senescence. The current desire for fiscal retrenchment at both the federal and state levels does not augur well for any major initiatives to reinvigorate the current regulatory environment.

Two major structural issues compound the problems stemming from the ineffectiveness of the current regulatory programs. The first is the fragmentation of agency responsibility, and the second is the apparent shortage of an adequate supply of beds. In many, if not most, states a facility is licensed and inspected by one agency, paid by a second agency, and assigned residents by a third.[74] This system almost ensures that homes with violations can continue to operate. In some cases the licensing and standard setting alone may be spread through several agencies. For example, in Pennsylvania, licensing and standard setting is carried out by one unit within the Department of Public Welfare, while approval for participation in the Medicare program is the responsibility of the Department of Health. Responsibility for approval with reference to fire safety is the responsibility of the Department of Labor and Industry.[75] Lack of interdepartmental communication may result in one agency trying to prod a facility to improve some aspect of its operation while another agency is increasing its reimbursement rate. Fragmentation of responsibility stemming from narrow jurisdictional boundaries has been noted as a factor hampering the effectiveness of the regulatory process in Illinois, Indiana,

Massachusetts, Minnesota, Oregon, Rhode Island, and Utah.[76] The results of the state health commissioner responsibility survey (noted in an earlier part of this chapter) indicated that while each of the 39 health departments responding had licensing and inspection responsibilities, only three had any rate-setting authority.* In the remaining 36 states, rate-setting authority is lodged in other agencies, usually the Department of Public Welfare. This Health-Welfare split is not a unique problem confronting only state government; a similar split and analogous problems exist at the federal level. Even when the licensing and rate-setting authority is lodged in a single state agency, as in New York, there often is minimal intraagency communication and coordination, thereby preventing a consolidated and consistent regulatory posture.[77]

The net result of this fragmentation of authority is that a major opportunity for prodding the industry toward higher levels of performance by tying reimbursement levels to patient-care needs and indexes of quality of care and quality of environment is lost.[78] Regulators are thus left with the choice of invoking relatively minor fines, which probably get passed on to private and public pay patients and are generally ineffective in encouraging change, or attempting to revoke a license, which is a lengthy, expensive, and often a seemingly futile process.

The second structural impediment, a limited supply of nursing home beds, prevents attempts at closing facilities that render unacceptable levels of care because there are no available beds to which to transfer the patients. In effect, unacceptable care is deemed to be better than no care at all. An inadequate supply of beds was noted as a reason for regulatory laxity in New York and Maryland, and as the primary cause of patient misplacement in Kentucky and New Hampshire.[79] The unavailability of alternatives to institutionalization clearly aggravates this problem. The certificate-of-need requirement may also act as a disincentive to the development of an adequate bed supply.†

IMPROVING THE PERFORMANCE OF THE LONG-TERM CARE SECTOR: OPTIONS, ISSUES, AND APPROACHES

Policy Options

It is evident from the material presented in the previous section that although the long-term care sector is already subject to extensive regu-

---

*The three state health departments with such responsibility were Arizona, New Jersey, and New York. In the case of New Jersey, the Health Department has yet to absorb this function from the Department of Institutions and Agencies.

†If the certificate-of-need process functions in the long-term sector in a manner analogous to that alleged by Salkaver and Bice in the acute care sector, then the net effect may be a cartel-induced shortage of beds.

lation at both the federal and the state levels, the regulatory efforts to date have not been successful in either improving the industry performance or ensuring that an acceptable level of care is provided to patients in long-term care facilities. This section sets forth several policy options that might lead to more effective regulatory mechanisms. Before one can suggest a number of specific policy alternatives, however, three crucial points merit consideration. They are: our limited economic capacity, the legal-political underpinnings of our democratic society, and the absence of a clearly superior ownership/control model.

The permissive environment of the 1960s, where sufficient funds appeared to be available to meet perceived social needs, has been replaced by the era of retrenchment in the 1970s. Government, at all levels, has been experiencing larger and larger deficits, and is beginning to realize that unlimited public borrowing and tax increases are neither permanent nor viable policies for meeting such deficits.

The era of retrenchment does not bode well for solutions that rely exclusively on more spending, especially in areas where public concern is not acute. Long-term care is such an area. Although indignant about recently exposed abuses, the body politic prefers to overlook the poor performance of the industry. Need for improvement may be acute, but of relatively low priority in the overall social perspective. Thus, options that focus only on increasing the funding for the current level of regulatory efforts are unacceptable.

Democratic societies are dependent on legal systems to preserve individual rights against the exercise of government power and the encroachment of government control over individual activity. Political ties and the need for broad-based support to successfully compete in the political arena are also attributes of our democratic society. Solutions that fail to recognize these facts are themselves doomed to failure. Until these issues are addressed directly as part of an analysis of our social/moral/legal fabric, they will continue to be problems that the long-term care sector must cope with but cannot remedy on its own.

The fact that the profit motive has a tendency to subjugate social desires and to emphasize private or corporate desires has led many individuals to believe that for-profit enterprises should be discouraged from entering the health field. However, nonprofit control, by and of itself, is not a solution to the perceived problem. It is incorrectly assumed that just because nonprofit corporations are prevented by law from distributing profits to shareholders, they are prevented from seeking and distributing "profits" through different channels. Within the acute care hospital sector, nonprofit control may have shifted the conventional distribution of profit primarily toward the physician, and to a lesser degree, the administrator and the remainder of the labor force. If the accrual of "profits" is recognized as the goal of all enterprises, then the policy issue becomes one of which groups in society should share in the profits, rather than whether profit making should be encouraged or tolerated. This assertion is buttressed by the fact that some evidence is available that indicates that within the long-term care sector, many proprietary facilities provide care at a level of quality comparable to voluntary facilities but at lower cost.[80] Thus, advocating a wholesale transformation of the industry in the direction of voluntary control does not appear to be either an effective or an efficient solution.

In light of these factors, five courses of action appear possible.

Option 1. Rescind the various regulatory programs and statutes and substitute market regulation for bureaucratic regulation.

Option 2. Accept the curent situation as the best that is possible given the current knowledge and financial constraints.

Option 3. Extend the current regulatory programs by identifying problem areas and promulgating additional rules and standards.

Option 4. Strengthen the existing regulatory mechanisms by streamlining the volume of regulatory requirements, devising strategies that will add "muscle" to the regulatory process and creating an environment where regulatory passivity will be minimized.

Option 5. Refocus the thrust of the regulatory programs from their current structure-process orientation to an outcome orientation and minimize the regulatory interventions in the day-to-day operation of long-term care facilities.

One additional option could have been proposed, namely, to declare the long-term care sector a public utility.[81] Public utility status would undoubtedly necessitate the creation of a new regulatory commission or agency at the federal level without reducing significantly the vast array of inspectors, auditors, accountants, and other professional and support personnel at the state level. Furthermore, public utility status, by and of itself, would not create new mechanisms or approaches to regulation. In effect, the industry already "enjoys" public utility status and may be more highly regulated than most public utilities. Consequently, declaring the industry a public utility appears to be a cosmetic rather than a substantive policy option.

No concrete evidence exists to support the contention that market regulation will be any more successful than bureaucratic regulation in guaranteeing that the providers of long-term care services will deliver quality care in an efficient manner. Competitive pressures would be absent in many geographical areas because nursing homes either enjoy local monopolies or can easily engage in cartel-like behavior, thus negating the presumed economic benefits of a perfectly competitive market. In the absence of substantial third-party payments, new capital may not flow into this sector. Prior to the mass infusion of Medicaid funds into the industry, both proprietary and voluntary interests exhibited a lack of interest in entering this market. While no major studies have investigated whether the infusion of substantial public payments is a cost-effective way to encourage economic efficiency via the perfectly competitive model, this author doubts whether such an approach could be supported at the political level or justified at the economic level.

Furthermore, the competitive approach is geared to ensuring profit maximization for the providers of care rather than quality of care maximization. Only if consumers are capable of judging the quality of the product and are concerned about the quality rather than the availability of the product, will quality considerations enter the provider's profit maximization function. The actual consumers of long-term care services are, by and large, not in a position to judge quality. Their judgment capabilities are hampered by the physical and mental deterioration that becomes acute at advanced ages, and by the fear of entering a new environment. Those who can attempt to judge quality, and who, in fact, are the real consumers of long-term care services, are the family, friends, or public guardians of the elderly and infirm. Social and economic pressures often encourage these consumers to attach much higher priority to removing those who require care from the home or community than to finding the best place for the one requiring institutionalization. The fact that nursing homes are, to a large extent, viewed as society's dumping ground for presumably used-up people practically ensures low attention to the quality of care provided.

Consequently, the first option does not appear to be a viable one. This conclusion is based primarily on social-moral considerations and could be advocated even in the face of economic evidence that the market approach would be less costly. It is one of the basic tenets of our society that some form of government intervention is justifiable to protect the health and safety of those individuals who cannot ensure such protection by their own initiatives.

Option two, the perpetuation of the status quo, is also an unacceptable one. Both the spirit and the letter of the law (conditions of participation/ standards) appear to be subject to major violations. It is questionable, both from a social and economic perspective, whether the output received under current conditions justifies the input extended. To accept option two as even a short-term goal is to permit the perpetuation of an ineffective and costly process.

The analysis of the factors contributing to the current regulatory failure do not provide one with any reason to advocate "more of the same" which, in effect, is option three. Recognizing the futility of the current regulatory program implies that option two is probably preferable to option three. It will entail lower resource expenditures and would probably yield the same end product with respect to patient care and industry performance.

Option four—strengthening and streamlining the existing regulatory process—appears to be a justified course of action in the short run. Our knowledge base and the current state of the art with respect to data systems in the long-term care field will not permit a successful revamping of the regulatory process (option five) within the next five or possibly ten years. Furthermore, attempts to strengthen the existing regulatory process provide an excellent opportunity to judge whether the political will exists to make regulation work.

Improving the Regulatory Process

The effectiveness of the current regulatory programs could be heightened by implementing five specific proposals. They are: eliminating the fragmentation in regulatory authority, directly linking the inspection/rate-setting processes, streamlining the volume of regulatory requirements, creating a role for the participation of external consumer groups in the current regulatory process, and exposing the process and results of regulation to public scrutiny.

Both inter- and intraagency fragmentation must be eliminated if the exercise of regulatory authority is to be effective. Assigning inspection and licensing responsibilities to the state health agency and rate-setting responsibilities to the state welfare agency creates an unnecessary gap that results in poor communication, and one that is not easily bridged in environments where agency rivalry is rife. The management literature is clear on the need for centralization of authority if the effective exercise of authority is desired. Creating an executive agency or committee to oversee and/or coordinate the regulatory powers of the health and welfare agencies is a possible solution to the problem. However, it is questionable whether day-to-day coordination can be achieved in this manner. A more effective approach appears to be the consolidation of the licensing-inspection and rate-setting functions in one agency.

The fact that the major expenditures for long-term care emanate from the welfare side suggests that the welfare agency be given the licensing-inspection role. However, the poor record achieved by welfare agencies in effecting desired levels of care in personal care homes and in the forerunners of the modern nursing homes does not inspire much confidence.[82] The proposal embodied in option five—to develop measures of quality of care and quality of life as the basis for regulatory action—raises the question of which of the two agencies (health or welfare) possesses the greater expertise in these areas. To the extent that such measures, when developed, are based on medical-nursing expertise, the health agency would appear to be the logical base for the consolidation of regulatory power. However, if social services and other welfare-related expertise is required to implement and analyze the proposed output measures, the welfare agency may be the logical site. In all probability, the skills required for constructing and interpreting outcome measures are possessed exclusively by neither agency. Thus, the choice will ultimately have to be made on other criteria. From our perspective, it makes no difference which agency absorbs the functions of the other as long as consolidation is achieved.

Once both functions are lodged in a single agency, steps should be taken to ensure that the rate-setting process includes rather than excludes the input derived from the inspection process. From a "table of organization" perspective, separate bureaus should be assigned the responsibility for the actual inspection and accounting duties. Both of these bureaus should report to a higher level of authority—assistant or deputy commissioner level—where the actual rate-setting process should be lodged.

While the analysis presented in this chapter focused exclusively on nursing homes, the fact remains that nursing homes are but one component of the long-term care industry. True coordination within the long-term care sector will not be achieved until the agency with regulatory responsibility for nursing homes also is given regulatory responsibility for specialized facilities (hospitals and other "health care" institutions) providing mental health care, and for institutions providing personal or domiciliary care.* The absence of a "continuous line of authority" practically guarantees the lack of policy coordination. This in turn is bound to result in patient misplacement.

Two phenomena illustrate this problem. Within the last few years, there has been a deliberate attempt to remove patients with mental health problems from mental hospitals and to return them to the "community." The reality behind this policy is that patients with serious mental disorders wind up in nursing homes that are ill-equipped to render care to them. Not only do such patients receive inappropriate care, but their presence in a facility often adversely affects the overall facility environment. Thus, health department officials must cope with a problem stemming from decisions made autonomously by the state mental health agency.

The regulations promulgated for the Supplemental Security Income Program, which is a major source of financing for personal or domiciliary care, appear to preclude any interface between low-level medical care and high-level congregate care, two basic elements in any long-term care program. Section 249D of Public Law 92-603 specifies that federal matching funds are not available for any portion of any payment by a state under Titles I, IV-A, X, XIV, or XVI of the Social Security Act for medical or remedial care, if such care is, or could be, provided under a state plan

----

*The survey of Health Commissioner authority (noted in the preceding section) indicated that only 17 of the responding 39 health departments had any jurisdiction over personal care or domiciliary care facilities in their state.

approved under Title XIX of the Social Security Act or by an institution certified under Title XIX. Federal regulations promulgated on November 29, 1973 (45 CFR 233.145c) define medical or remedial services provided in an institutional setting as any service beyond room, board, and laundry.

From a structural perspective, jurisdiction over long-term care services appears to be dispersed over a wide range of state and federal agencies, thus preventing both the establishment of unified policy goals and the analysis of long-term care problems from an industry perspective. Until a program rather than a functional focus is adopted, and agency and departmental boundaries are readjusted to coincide with this new perspective, the effectiveness of any regulatory efforts will be greatly diminished.

Once agency reorganization focused on merging regulatory authority within a single area of responsibility is accomplished, steps must be taken to directly link the inspection/rate-setting processes. Tremendous regulatory leverage is lost if rate setting is viewed solely as a mechanism for reimbursement for expenditures incurred upon the receipt of the appropriate vouchers. The rate-setting process should not only ensure adequate reimbursement,* but should also be used as a mechanism to improve both operating efficiency and quality of care/quality of life, and to direct individuals' quest for profits along socially desired lines. If such an approach is adopted, heavy fines and license revocation will no longer appear to be the only devices for insuring compliance with regulatory directives. An equally powerful mechanism, which does not rely exclusively on the "stick" but also offers a "carrot" for good performance, is available to help achieve desired goals.

The studies reviewed above indicate that cost controls may have been an effective regulatory measure. However, input intensity—one aspect of quality of care—has been sacrificed in the process. A reimbursement mechanism should be developed to link the inspection/rate-setting processes but also to insure that economies are not realized at the expense of socially desired quality levels.[83] Briefly, we propose that per diem reimbursement should be a function of four factors: facility grouping and the establishment of dollar ceilings within each group; degree of resource utilization (occupancy rate); patient assessment and classification into health status categories; and facility evaluation. Evaluating and reimbursing a facility through a grouping mechanism, where performance is compared with that of peer group facilities, should introduce an element of competition, which, in the absence of collusion, will lead to an improvement in operating efficiency.

---

*It is crucial that the set reimbursement rate be adequate, in an accounting sense, to cover the total cost of care that is desired. Unless this precept is adhered to, the resultant quality level will never be achieved. Providers of care cannot be expected to subsidize quality. At best, they will provide the level of care that they are paid to, and no more.

The novel aspect of the reimbursement proposal is the requirement for developing a patient health status index for each facility that reflects quality of care/quality of life considerations. The derivation of the patient health status index should be based on data derived from a periodic patient and facility assessment process that should include an extensive patient-oriented medical/social/behavioral evaluation and a concomitant assessment of the facility's performance in meeting the patient's needs. Based on the data generated by this process, patients would be assigned to designated health status categories. The sum of the number of patients in each category times a predetermined weight will yield an institution-specific health status index.

This index then forms the basis for adjusting a traditional prospective reimbursement rate for the actuarially determined cost of providing care to patient cohorts with health status index scores above or below the group average. The nature of the adjustment can be illustrated by the following hypothetical example. Assume that it costs X dollars to provide non-administrative care to health status category Y, which is the mean health status category for all facilities in a given grouping schema. Further assume that the industry-wide costs of unit increases or decreases (Z) from the mean health status category have been ascertained by econometric analysis, and that a given facility has a health status index 40 percent above the mean. The facility's final reimbursement rate is determined by segregating its preliminary per diem reimbursement rate into administrative and non-administrative operating costs on the basis of historical evidence; multiplying the nonadministrative costs by $1.40Z$; and adding the adjusted nonadministrative to the administrative costs, thereby obtaining the total reimbursement rate. Thus, higher reimbursement is received if the index value implies a need for and existence of an intensive level of care, and lower reimbursement is received for providing lower levels of care.

It is further proposed that states could and should build in "profit" factors into those areas that enhance the patient care and environment aspects of the facility, such as patient activities and rehabilitation programs. Such avenues for profit making are clearly of greater social value than the current approaches to facility cost-reimbursement that cater to real estate interests and acquiesce in the accrual of relatively high profits by non "arms-length" sale and/or leasing arrangements that artificially inflate depreciation and interest charges.[84]

A third way in which the regulatory process can be strengthened is by streamlining the volume of regulatory requirements. Current regulatory directives affect practically every aspect of a nursing home's operations. Regulatory requirements are especially detailed for facilities rendering skilled nursing care. For example, experience and educational background requirements exist for practically all the professional and nonprofessional staff. Staff salaries account for over 50 percent of a facility's operating costs. Specified construction and physical environment requirements also influence both operating and capital costs. Evidence is required on the effectiveness of each regulatory directive and its relationship to quality of care. Research should be undertaken to clarify these points, and the findings should serve as the basis for the suggested streamlining.

A fourth approach to strengthening the regulatory process is to develop mechanisms for external participation in inspections, and to include provisions for such activities in the Medicare/Medicaid conditions of participation/standards. Although the impetus for this proposal comes from the general consumerism movement,[85] its thrust is directed at retarding or reversing the presumed natural slide of regulatory agencies into patterns of "apathy" and "senility." Not only can consumer groups relieve the pressure on state inspection teams by assuming some of the inspection responsibilities, but they also can enhance the entire inspection process by bringing a new and nonclinical perspective to the inspection process. Furthermore, their presence in any facility on a semiregular basis may prove to be therapeutic for the facility's residents who generally have minimal contact with the "outside" world. Local voluntary associations in the field of the aged and associations of retired individuals, such as the association of retired teachers, would be able to identify with facility residents and to assess the quality of the environment better than other consumer groups. If such groups could be induced to assume facility visitation responsibilities on at least a quarterly basis, they would be in a position to file annual reports that would be considered part of the inspection document and to request special state investigations where they felt that major violations existed. Hopefully, the involvement of such local groups would help to: (a) impart an aura of a "community asset" to nursing homes similar to that enjoyed by most public schools and local hospitals, (b) involve local groups as volunteers or regular visitors in nursing homes, and (c) boost the morale of facility staff by creating the opportunity for recognition and appreciation.[86] The extra costs arising from external participation should be considered as part of the total inspection borne completely by the federal government under the provisions of Section 249B of P.L. 92-603, which provides federal payments to states under Medicaid for compensation of inspectors responsible for maintaining compliance with federal standards.

A fifth proposal, also intended to prevent passivity on the part of regulatory agencies, is to require that all regulatory activities be opened to public scrutiny, and that all regulatory decisions be subject to public disclosure. Copies of facility inspection reports, including the external group evaluation, should be disseminated by the responsible state agency to the local press and to interested civic and consumer groups, and should be displayed in a position of prominence in each facility. Failure to display the most current report should constitute a violation of the state's rules and standards. Authority for such disclosures appears to exist under the provisions of Section 299D of P.L. 92-603; however, few efforts appear to have been undertaken to date in this area. All hearings connected with the licensing process and with attempts to invoke sanctions for noncompliance should be announced and open to the public. To facilitate this proposal, it is suggested that Medicare conditions of participation and Medicaid standards be revised to require public accountability and public disclosure of nonconfidential material.

Improving the Regulatory Environment

In addition to the five specific proposals for enhancing the effectiveness of the regulatory process, a number of additional suggestions are offered for directly improving the regulatory environment. These suggestions include eliminating the barriers to entry created by inadequate reimbursement levels and the certificate-of-need process, supporting alternatives to institutionalization, federalizing the Medicaid program, abandoning the exclusive reliance on the medical model as a guide for regulatory standards, and facilitating the required knowledge generation process.

As noted in the preceding section, one factor hampering the effectiveness of the regulatory process is the inadequate supply of "conforming" beds. New entry into the industry appears to be effectively blocked. Two explanations exist for this phenomenon. First, reimbursement rates may be inadequate to ensure a "fair" profit, and second, the certificate-of-need process may have become a tool to enhance the interests of current providers of care at the expense of potential providers. The brief discussion of the proposed linking of the patient assessment-reimbursement processes noted the need for the determination of actuarially fair levels of reimbursement. It should be quite evident that rate setting must be based on the cost of providing the desired level of care in an economically efficient manner. To set rates based on any other criteria is to invite noncompliance. To date, most state rate-setting agencies have not received the necessary financial allocations to permit such rate setting. The requirement of a cost-related rate-setting formula effective July 1978 as specified in Section 249 of P.L. 92-603 provides the necessary legislative initiative to redress the problem of inadequate reimbursement levels. However, the problems stemming from inadequate reimbursement will not be effectively addressed unless the word "related" is interpreted as mandating full payment for care rendered in an efficient manner at levels specified in the Medicare conditions of participation and the Medicaid standards.*

---

*The fiscal ramifications of this suggestion are addressed as part of the discussion of proposed revisions in the Medicare/Medicaid programs.

Once the adequacy of reimbursement levels is assured, the certificate-of-need process must be carefully examined. If it acts as a barrier to needed new entry, it should be revised or scrapped. It is clearly inconsistent to devise regulatory programs whose intent is to reduce cost but whose effect is a cartel-induced shortage, and to simultaneously lament the unavailability of an adequate supply of beds.

The absence of alternatives to institutional care forces the institutionalization of people who could remain in the community if specialized ambulatory care programs and supportive programs such as home care, homemaker services, meals-on-wheels, visiting nurse service, special transportation programs, and congregate living arrangements were available. Such programs would presumably be less costly than institutionalization, would enable people requiring some supportive care to avoid the psychological trauma that often accompanies institutionalization, and should minimize the need for the construction of additional nursing home beds. The availability of alternatives to institutional care would also greatly enhance the overall performance of the long-term care sector by providing a more appropriate match between many patients' needs and services provided. By providing extra bed capacity, the availability of noninstitutional care would remove one of the barriers to the effective exercise of regulatory authority.

The limited coverage available for nursing home care under private health insurance plans and under the Medicare program leaves Medicaid as the dominant source of third-party payments in the nursing home field. In some states Medicaid payments account for 90 percent of nursing home revenue. Two aspects of the Medicaid program adversely affect the industry's performance and indirectly hamper regulatory effectiveness. These two aspects are the ''double jeopardy element'' introduced by the matching fund principle, and the uneven state commitment to finance and supervise their Medicaid programs.

Due to inadequate tax revenue, many states have been forced to reduce or temporarily freeze their overall contributions to their Medicaid programs.[87] However, a reduction in a state's contribution is matched by a reduction in the federal contribution, thus leading to a greater total reduction. In effect, changes in local economic conditions lead to a reduction in financing and ultimately in the quality of care provided. Decisions on quality of care provided should be made on a national rather than local level. The vast majority of nursing home residents are above 62 years of age. A national program, Social Security, was enacted to provide these people with financial substance during their retirement years. And yet when, in retirement, they require long-term care, the federal government appears to be abrogating the commitment inherent in the Social Security legislation by shifting the responsibility for the amount and quality of care provided to the states.

Equity considerations demand a uniform level of social services, yet under the Medicaid program, no such uniformity in state financing exists. The maximum per diem rate for skilled nursing care under the New Jersey Medicaid program is $28, while the maximum under the New York State program is approximately $75. Although Section 249B of P.L. 92-603 provides for 100 percent federal payment for compensation of inspectors responsible for maintaining compliance with federal nursing home standards, it does not provide compensating funds to the providers of care to overcome reductions in or low levels of state reimbursement and so insure that quality of care is not adversely affected. It makes little sense to promulgate national standards and guidelines and to expect adherence to them unless adequate payment for providing the required care is also insured.

The 1972 revisions in the Social Security Act (P.L. 92-603) amend Section 1811 of the act to include the disabled in addition to the aged. Disability connotes an element of permanency; long-term care entails the provision of therapeutic, rehabilitative, and custodial care to individuals who have chronic conditions. Chronicity also connotes an element of permanence. To overcome the problems stemming from the matching fund process and from the lack of uniformity in funding across states, it is proposed that both the initiative and responsibility for financing long-term care services be removed from the state level and lodged at the federal level. State responsibility for the licensing, inspection, and disbursement of reimbursement funds would be maintained under the current proposal.

Providing for a new element in the Medicaid program that would merely compensate for state fiscal difficulties would still leave the initiative for providing leadership in the long-term care policy realm with the states. Such leadership has been displayed in relatively few states. Even in the absence of the matching funds problem, it seems that the Medicaid program has not been a success. It is an interesting social experiment that highlighted the unwillingness or inability of most state goverments to rise to the occasion and provide leadership in the realm of adequate social services to the needy.

As noted in the official legislative document, P.L. 93-641 (National Health Planning and Resources Development Act of 1974) is "an act to amend the Public Health Service Act to assure the development of a national health policy." Under Section 1501 of P.L. 93-641, the Secretary of Health, Education, and Welfare is mandated to devise national health planning policy. Adequate financing and provision of long-term care services should clearly be part of any national health policy.

In developing national health policy for long-term care, attention must be given to the implicit approach embodied in the Medicare/Medicaid regulations and to an evaluation of the effectiveness of that approach. Prior to the enactment of the Medicare/Medicaid legislation, nursing home care was considered part of the social welfare system.[88] Medicare and Medicaid have cast long-term care in the medical model. The inappropriateness of this model for all long-term care facilities has been widely recognized, but has not yet led to any changes in our approach to regulating long-term care facilities.[89]

Long-term care services should be reoriented toward social-health needs. Patients with chronic conditions need psychosocial services, such as sensory awareness, as well as educational, creative, and religious activities. These services strengthen the self-image of patients so that they believe that they are a vital part of society, not an unwanted burden. Such programs often determine whether a long-term care patient will recover or regress, but are least recognized by the medical model.[90] This is particularly true for the must underserved and neglected patients within the long-term care sector—those with mental disabilities. In the medical model, if complex nursing procedures are not needed, the patient is not deemed to require skilled care. The psychopharmaceutical revolution has made possible the wholesale dumping of confused, elderly patients from state hospitals into nursing homes. These patients require a vast array of treatment modalities, including resocialization and remotivation, elements that are not central to the medical model. As reimbursement is currently pegged to facility level (SNF vs ICF), higher payments are available exclusively for those requiring or supposedly receiving skilled care. The lower reimbursement paid for intermediate care may be adequate to cover room and board expenses but not the provision of psychosocial services. As a result, such services are not provided.

It appears to be time for the pendulum to swing away from the medical-nursing model back toward the social welfare model. The social welfare model in a modern context, however, would emphasize psychosocial rather than traditional welfare needs. The acute care, medically oriented institution should be included as part of the long-term care spectrum, but only as a small part, and with strong ties to the acute care hospital sector. The model long-term care facilty should contain housing and social care as the basic component, with medical support provided internally or purchased externally as required. By and large, nursing homes have done a poor job in providing medical and nursing care. As an alternative to regarding medical services as the basis of care in long-term care facilities, policymakers might turn their attention to mechanisms that would enable these facilites to purchase specialized professional services from external groups. Providers of care should have wide latitude in combining various inputs or services to produce an acceptable level of care and environment. As long as output levels are socially acceptable, little attention need be given to the types and quantities of inputs used. We propose that, in the long run (when a sufficient knowledge base is available), regulatory review be based primarily on *outcome measures*. Attention should be directed only to those structural elements that directly relate to patient safety and to those process measures that have been shown to have a direct relationship to quality considerations and to be cost-effective.

To date, we have extremely limited knowledge of the elements that contribute to quality of life and quality of care—in a psychosocial rather than medical context—in the long-term care setting. A major research program is clearly called for in this area. A team of researchers at the Rush-Presbyterian-St. Luke's Medical Center in Chicago, in conjunction with the Medicus Systems Corporation, are already conducting some interesting research in this area.[91] Recognizing that long-term care must entail an active effort to rehabilitate and to restore the aged or chronically ill individual, and that any evaluation of the care process must focus on patient welfare, they developed a comprehensive methodology for the evaluation of quality of life and care in long-term care facilities. Their quality evaluation system is based on two sets of scaled measures. One set of 40 scales measures the quality of life and care provided by the facility. The other set of 28 scales measures the individual residents' needs for care. Scores on these scales are computed from data collected during facility surveys and patient reviews using highly structured survey instruments.

Resident needs, which are summarized in a need index, are based on the assessment of eight factors: basic physical competence, self-care competence, special nursing needs, emotional competence, social competence, verbal competence, spatial competence, and perceptions of the facility. The facility quality profile, summarized in a quality index, is based on measures of: enriched personalized environment, staff-resident relationship, involvement in activities, physical plant, personal services, administrative and support services, rehabilitation and restorative care, and health care services. In addition to these two indexes, two other measures are proposed. The first, focusing on the resident, is a set of matching scores, where each matching score is a ratio measure relating the resident's score on a specific need criterion to the facility's scores on a subset of the quality criteria most relevant to meeting that specific need of the resident. The second is simply the percentage of residents in a random sample from a facility's census whose matching scores equal or exceed distribution-dependent cutoff points (which are one standard deviation below the mean). Taken together, the matching scores and cutoff points provide a means of assessing the relative degree to which an individual's needs are met by the facility in which he has been placed.

Additional efforts paralleling the Rush-Presbyterian-St. Luke's Medical Center/Medicus Systems Corporation/Illinois Department of Public Health studies, and proposing new approaches for defining and quantifying quality of life-quality of care measures are clearly needed. Some interesting research on quality of care assessment in the acute health care sector has recently been completed that investigated variation in the assessment of quality of care as a function of the method used to measure it.[92] The results, which indicate that different methods produce substantially different results, raise a major point that must also be considered in developing quality measures.

A complementary need is the development and implementation of computerized information systems. Even the most valid information about quality is of little value to regulatory agencies unless the means are available to process it, store it, retrieve it, and apply it to specific decision-making tasks. Whereas Section 235 of P.L. 92-603 provides federal payments to states under Medicaid for the installation and operation of information retrieval systems,* very little progress appears to have been made in this regard.[93]

Interest Group Position and Time Frame

The changes in the regulatory process and environment noted in the previous two subsections are prerequisites or corequisites for implementing options 4 and 5 presented in the beginning of this section. These ten policy initiatives can be summarized as follows:

1. Eliminate fragmentation of regulatory responsibility.
2. Link the inspection/rate-setting processes.
3. Streamline the volume of existing regulatory requirements.
4. Create a role for the participation of external (consumer) groups in the regulatory process.
5. Expose the process and results of regulation to public scrutiny.
6. Eliminate barriers to entry.
7. Support alternatives to institutionalization.
8. Federalize the Medicaid program.
9. Shift the regulatory orientation from a medical to a psychosocial model.
10. Facilitate the required knowledge generation process to enable reglation on an outcome rather than a structure-process basis.

Steps can be taken immediately to implement or follow up on each of these items. Legislation will be required to implement the first and eighth suggestions; the remaining policy initiatives can be implemented by revising

---

*Section 235 provides for federal payment of 90 percent of the cost of design, development, and installation of an information system (up to a maximum of $150,000 each year) and of 75 percent of the operating costs. Approval of the secretary is required for the receipt of such payments.

the existing regulations and/or appropriating funds to support the required efforts.

Efforts were made to obtain the views of the two major associations of providers of long-term care on the recommended policy initiatives. The American Association of Homes for the Aging (AAHA) represents the nonprofit providers of care and the American Health Care Association (AHCA) is regarded as the spokesman for the for-profit providers of care.* In general, the AAHA would support most of the ten policy initiatives.† AAHA opposes dropping the certificate-of-need requirement because they fear that some "undesirable" proprietary groups will enter the field.‡ The group has also expressed its reservations with the suggestion for federalizing the Medicaid program into a Medicare-type program; its reservations are based on the premise that such a program will have too much of a hospital focus. However, AAHA does agree that mechanisms must be found to encourage entry and to unite all sources of third-party payments into a single funding mechanism.

The AHCA position is also supportive of most of the recommended policy initiatives. They did feel, however, that consumers should not participate in the inspection process unless they are specifically trained for this function, and question whether the input received from consumers would be truly objective. While the AHCA recognizes the problems inherent in the current Medicaid program, they feel that policy initiative 8 is impractical at this point in time.

It is quite obvious that some of the recommended policy initiatives are controversial and require further thought and analysis prior to implementation. Eliminating the fragmentation of regulatory responsibility and federalizing the Medicaid program are two recommendations which fall into this category. Another recommendation—shifting the nature of regulation from a structure-process orientation to an outcome orientation—can not be acted upon immediately because the required knowledge base is not available. Consequently, these three recommendations become "long-run" options.

Efforts should be made immediately to lay the groundwork for linking the inspection and rate-setting processes, streamlining the volume of regulatory requirements, eliminating barriers to entry, supporting alternatives to institutionalization, and shifting the regulatory orientation from a medi-

---

*The membership roster of AHCA does include nonprofit providers.

†Officials of AAHA and AHCA were informed of the specific policy recommendations presented in this study. However, they did not have access to the entire report. Consequently, support for any recommended course of action implies support in a general rather than a specific sense.

‡The author feels that any desired screening can be accomplished through the licensing mechanism.

cal to a psychosocial model. Although we recognize that some time must elapse between the espousal of these policy initiatives and their ultimate implementation, they remain "short-run" options.

Policy initiatives 4 and 5—creating a role for the participation of external consumer groups in the regulatory process and exposing the process and results of regulation to public scrutiny—can be implemented within a brief period of time. Thus, they and the research agenda required to implement policy options 3 and 10 are the recommendations that can be implemented within the "immediate" period.

Conclusion

It is quite evident that it is extremely difficult to develop and administer effective regulations. In part this is because regulation runs counter to provider self-interest. However, the major problem appears to be that we know less than we should like to about the entity we are attempting to regulate—the quality of long-term care services. In the absence of the required technical knowledge, no regulator can easily support new regulatory initiatives.

Much that is wrong today in the health sector derives from the fact that the structure of the health industry provides the wrong incentives.[94] Within the long-term care sector, regulation has failed to correct this state because it is divorced from the natural mechanism for offering incentives for good performance—reimbursement—and it is based primarily on the inputs associated with the acute care medical model. The proposals presented in this paper seek to correct these and the other problems that detract from the effectiveness of the regulatory effort. The adoption of the proposed policy initiatives entails, in a sense, the ultimate trial of regulation. If a system such as the one proposed in this paper does not work, then one is led a good way toward the conclusion that no regulation will work and that other alternatives best be initiated. However, it should be noted that the industry power that has been manifest in attempts to thwart regulatory directives will be no less vigorously displayed in blocking any attempts at directing the industry's performance.

The suggested course of action is clearly a costly one. If it is implemented, the long-term care sector will absorb a greater proportion of the gross national product than it does today. Such a prescription is bound to elicit serious objections in an era where official policy appears to be directed toward a reduction in federal spending and responsibility. However, in the final analysis, the problems of the long-term care sector cannot be effectively solved at other levels of government. We must either agree to commit a greater proportion of our resources to this sector of the health field or lower our sights and accept the status quo.

NOTES

1. U.S., Congress, Senate, Special Committee on Aging, *Nursing Home Care in the United States: Failure in Public Policy* (Washington, D.C.: Government Printing Office, 1974), p. iii.

2. For a detailed discussion of these problem areas see Hirsch S. Ruchlin et al., "The Long-Term Care Marketplace: An Analysis of Deficiencies and Potential Reform by Means of Incentive Reimbursement," *Medical Care* 13, no. 12 (1975), pp. 979–91.

3. U.S., Congress, Special Committee on Aging, *Nursing Home Care*, pp. iii–iv.

4. Robert K. Byron et al., "A Model Act for the Regulation of Long-Term Health Care Facilities," *Harvard Journal on Legislation* 8, no. 11 (1970), p. 56.

5. U.S., Congress, Special Committee on Aging, *Nursing Home Care*, p. 51.

6. Elias S. Cohen, *Long-Term Care: A Challenge to Concerted Legal Techniques* (Philadelphia: Department of Community Medicine, School of Medicine, University of Pennsylvania, 1973), pp. 19–22. Mimeographed.

7. Paul W. MacAvoy, ed., *The Crisis of the Regulatory Commissions* (New York: W. W. Norton, 1970), p. viii; Clark C. Havighurst, "Public Utility Regulation for Hospitals: The Relevance of Experience in Other Regulated Industries," Reprint No. 17 (Washington, D.C.: American Enterprise Institute, 1973), pp. 10, 13, 18; Patrick O'Donoghue, *Evidence About the Effects of Health Care Regulation* (Denver: Spectrum Research, Inc., 1974), p. 123; and Roger G. Noll, "The Consequences of Public Utility Regulation of Hospitals," in National Academy of Sciences, Institute of Medicine, *Controls on Health Care* (Washington, D.C.: National Academy of Sciences, 1975), p. 33.

8. Robert E. Schlenker, *Public Utility Regulation of the Health Care Delivery System—Lessons from Other Regulated Industries* (Minneapolis: Inter Study, 1973), p. 5. Mimeographed.

9. Mark Green and Ralph Nader, "Economic Regulation vs. Competition: Uncle Sam The Monopoly Man," *Yale Law Journal* 82, no. 5 (1973), p. 882.

10. Lawrence J. White, "Quality Regulation When Prices Are Regulated," *The Bell Journal of Economics and Management Science* 5, no. 2 (1974), pp. 425–36.

11. Marver H. Bernstein, *Regulating Business by Independent Commission* (Princeton: Princeton University Press, 1955), pp. 155–56; and Louis L. Jaffe, "The Effective Limits of the Administrative Process: A Reevaluation," *Harvard Law Review* 67, no. 7 (1954), pp. 902–32.

12. George J. Stigler, "The Theory of Economic Regulation," *The Bell Journal of Economics and Management Science* 2, no. 1 (1971), pp. 3–21.

13. Richard A. Posner, "Theories of Economic Regulation," *The Bell Journal of Economics and Management Science* 5, no. 2 (1974), pp. 335–58.

14. John R. Baldwin, *The Regulatory Agency and the Public Corporation: The Canadian Air Transport Industry* (Cambridge, Mass.: Ballinger Publishing Co., 1975), ch. 1; and James Q. Wilson, "The Dead Hand of Regulation," *The Public Interest*, no. 25 (Fall 1971), pp. 39–58.

15. Wilson, "The Dead Hand," pp. 47–48.

16. Bernstein, *Regulating Business*, ch. 2; Merle Fainsod, "Some Reflections on the Nature of the Regulatory Process," in Library of Congress, Legislative Reference Service, *Separation of Powers and the Independent Agencies: Cases and Selected Readings* (Washington, D.C.: Government Printing Office, 1970), pp. 470–96; and Emmette S. Redford, "Perspectives for the Study of Government Regulation," *The Midwest Journal of Political Science* 6, no. 2 (1962), pp. 1–18.

17. Lee Loevinger, "Regulation and Competition as Alternatives," *The Antitrust Bulletin* 11, nos. 1 and 2 (1966), p. 137.

18. Robert M. Ball, "Background of Regulation in Health Care," in National Academy of Sciences, Institute of Medicine, pp. 21–22.

19. Anne R. Somers, *Hospital Regulation: The Dilemma of Public Policy* (Princeton: Industrial Relations Section, Princeton University, 1969), p. 16.

20. Stuart Altman and Joseph Eichenholz, "Control of Hospital Cost Under the Economic Stabilization Program," *Federal Register* 39, no. 60 (1974), Appendix to Subpart R, Table 3.

21. Paul B. Ginsburg, "Price Controls and Hospital Costs" (paper presented at the 101st annual meeting of the American Public Health Association, San Francisco, Nov. 1974), Table 1.

22. Paul B. Ginsburg, "Price Controls and Hospital Costs" (paper presented at the 87th annual meeting of the American Economic Association, San Francisco, Dec. 1974), p. 26. The theoretical model of hospital behavior developed by Ginsburg leads him to hypothesize that ESP should have led to an *increase* in mean stay.

23. Ralph E. Berry, "Evaluation of Prospective Hospital Reimbursement in New York" (paper presented at the 88th annual meeting of the American Economic Association, Dallas, Texas, Dec. 1975), p. 16.

24. For a discussion of some of the effects of New York's stringent fiscal controls, see Alan L. Appelbaum, "New York City Hospitals: The Financial Crunch," *Hospitals* 50, no. 2 (1976), pp. 59–62.

25. Lewin and Associates, Inc., *Nationwide Survey of State Health Regulations*, Document No. PB-236600 (Springfield, Virginia: National Technical Information Service, 1974), p. 31.

26. Lewin and Associates, *An Analysis of State and Regional Health Regulation*, Part I: Report of the Study, Document No. PB-240966 (Springfield, Virginia: National Technical Information Service, 1974), pp. 2–9.

27. Case Studies in Prospective Reimbursement for the Social Security Administration: Grant 5-P16-HS 00472 (NCHSRD). Arthur D. Little, "The Prospective Reimbursement Program of Blue Cross of Northeast Ohio" (1973); "The Prospective Reimbursement Program of Blue Cross of Southwest Ohio" (1973); "The Prospective Reimbursement Program of Blue Cross of Northeast Pennsylvania" (1973); "The Prospective Reimbursement Program of Connecticut Blue Cross" (1974); "The Prospective Reimbursement Programs in the State of Colorado" (1974); "The Prospective Hospital Rate Review Program for Blue Cross of Wisconsin Payments to Hospitals" (1974); K. G. Bauer, "The Combined Budget Review and Formula Approach to Prospective Reimbursement by the Blue Cross of Western Pennsylvania" (1974); and K. G. Bauer and A. V. Clark, "Budget Reviews and Prospective Rate Setting for Rhode Island Hospitals" (1974); "New York: The Formula Approach to Prospective Reimbursement" (1974); "The Indiana Controlled Charges System" (1974); "The New Jersey Budget Review Program" (1974).

28. W. Thomas Berriman et al., "Capital Projects," *Topics in Health Care Financing* 2, no. 2 (1975), Appendix B. The 29 states with certificate-of-need legislation were: Arizona, Arkansas, California, Colorado, Connecticut, Florida, Georgia, Hawaii, Illinois, Kansas, Kentucky, Maryland, Massachusetts, Michigan, Minnesota, Montana, Nevada, New Jersey, New York, North Dakota, Oklahoma, Oregon, Rhode Island, South Carolina, South Dakota, Tennessee, Texas, Virginia, and Washington.

29. Berriman et al., *Capital Projects*, Appendix C. These states are: Alabama, Alaska, Arkansas, Colorado, Delaware, Florida, Georgia, Hawaii, Idaho, Indiana, Iowa, Kentucky, Louisiana, Maine, Maryland, Michigan, Minnesota, Mississippi, Missouri, Montana, Nebraska, Nevada, New Hampshire, New Jersey, New Mexico, New York, North Carolina, North Dakota, Ohio, Oklahoma, Oregon, Pennsylvania, South Carolina, Utah, Virginia, Vermont, Washington, Wisconsin, and Wyoming.

30. William J. Curran et al., "Government Intervention on Increase," *Hospitals* 49, no. 10 (1975), pp. 59–60; Lewin and Associates, *An Analysis of State and Regional Health Regulation*, pp. 2–21.

31. Ibid., "Government Intervention," p. 58.

32. Clark C. Havighurst. "Regulation of Health Institutions." in National Academy of Sciences. Institute of Medicine. p. 81.

33. William J. Curran. "A Severe Blow to Hospital Planning: Certificate-of-Need Declared Unconstitutional." *New England Journal of Medicine* 288. no. 14 (1973). p. 723: and Macro Systems, Inc.. *The Certificate-of-Need Experience*. Vol. I: Summary Report (Silver Spring: Macro Systerms, Inc.. 1974). p. 9. Mimeographed. The program referred to in the Curran article is the North Carolina Program. and it is the only one that has been repealed to date.

34. David S. Salkever and Thomas W. Bice. "The Impact of Certificate-of-Need Controls on Hospital Investment." *Milbank Memorial Fund Quarterly* 54. no. 2 (1976). p. 26.

35. William Worthington and Laurens H. Silver. "Regulation of Quality of Care in Hospitals: The Need for Change." *Law and Contemporary Problems* 35. no. 2 (1970). p. 309.

36. Ibid.. p. 310.

37. "H.E.W. Must Answer Subpoena on Hospital Certifying Report." *New York Times*. Nov. 10. 1975. p. 36.

38. Milton I. Roemer. A. Thaer Moustafa. and Carl E. Hopkins. "A Proposed Hospital Quality Index: Hospital Death Rates Adjusted for Case Severity." *Health Services Research* 3. no. 2 (1968). p. 115.

39. "Audits Reducing Shortcomings in Hospitals." *New York Times*. Jan. 29. 1976. p. 24.

40. See Lowell E. Bellin. "PSRO-Quality Control? Or Gimmickry?" *Medical Care* 12. no. 12 (1974). pp. 1012–18.

41. "Most Doctors Reluctant to Report Incompetent Work by Their Colleagues." *New York Times*. Jan. 29. 1976. p. 24.

42. Harold A. Cohen. "State Rate Regulation." in National Academy of Sciences. Institute of Medicine. p. 135: and A. J. G. Priest. "Possible Adaptation of Public Utility Concepts in the Health Care Field." *Law and Contemporary Problems* 35. no. 4 (1970). pp. 839–48.

43. U.S.. Department of Health. Education. and Welfare. Audit Agency—Region V. "Report on Audit of Skilled Nursing Home Services Provided Under the Medicaid Program. Title XIX of the Social Security Act. State of Indiana." Audit Control No. 05-50002. June 27. 1974. pp. 28–32. Mimeographed: U.S.. Department of Health. Education. and Welfare. Audit Agency—Region IV. "Audit of Administration of the Skilled Nursing Home Program. Title XIX of the Social Security Act. As Administered by the Commonwealth of Kentucky." Audit Control No. 04-40152. July 24. 1973. p. 19. Mimeographed: U.S.. Department of Health. Education. and Welfare. Audit Agency—Region I. "Review of the Commonwealth of Massachusetts Certification Program for Skilled Nursing Facilities." Audit Control No. 40047-01. January 23. 1974. p. 5. Mimeographed: and U.S.. Department of Health. Education. and Welfare. Audit Agency—Region I. "Review of Nursing Home Operations Under Title XIX of the Social Security Act and the Categorical Public Assistance Programs As Administered by the State of Rhode Island." Audit Control No 40008-01. July 12. 1973. pp. 6–7. Mimeographed. Due to limited access to HEW audit reports. the enumeration of states with operating deficiencies in their nursing home programs is not necessarily complete.

44. Indiana Report. pp. 28. 30.

45. U.S.. Department of Health. Education. and Welfare. Audit Agency—Region I. "Review of Selected Aspects of Skilled Nursing Facility and Intermediate Care Facility Level of Care Operations Under Title XIX—Social Security Act. As Administered by the State of New Hampshire." Audit Control No. 40077-01. June 7. 1974. p. 9. Mimeographed.

46. Rhode Island Report. p. 23: and U.S.. Department of Health. Education. and Welfare. Audit Agency—Region X. "Report on Audit of the Medicaid Skilled Nursing Facilities Program Under Title XIX. Social Security Act. Administered by the State of Idaho." Audit Control No. 40014-10. December 19. 1973. p. 11. Mimeographed.

47. U.S., Department of Health, Education, and Welfare, Audit Agency—Region V, "Report on Audit of Selected Aspects of Skilled Nursing Home Care Provided Under the Medical Assistance Program, State of Minnesota," Audit Control No. 05-40085, March 28, 1974, p. 17. Mimeographed.

48. U.S., Department of Health, Education, and Welfare, Audit Agency—Region I, "Review of Selected Aspects of Skilled and Intermediate Care Nursing Home Operations Under Titles XVI and XIX of the Social Security Act, As Administered by the State of Maine," Audit Control No. 40012-01, December 7, 1973, p. 7. Mimeographed; Kentucky Report, p. 11; Idaho Report, p. 22; and U.S., Department of Health, Education, and Welfare, Audit Agency—Region V, "Report on Audit of Nursing Home Services Provided Under Title XIX of the Social Security Act, State of Illinois," Audit Control No. 05-50012, November 19, 1974, p. 4. Mimeographed.

49. U.S., Congress, Senate, Special Committee on Aging, Subcommittee on Long-Term Care, *Doctors in Nursing Homes: The Shunned Responsibility*, Supporting Paper No. 3 (Washington, D.C.: Government Printing Office, 1975), p. 331.

50. U.S., Department of Health, Education, and Welfare, Audit Agency—Region IV, "Report on Audit of Georgia State Department of Human Resources Administration of State-Operated Skilled Nursing Care Facilities Under the Medical Assistance Program," Audit Control No. 04-50150, August 22, 1974, p. 6. Mimeographed; Illinois Report, p. 6; Indiana Report, p. 12; U.S., Department of Health, Education, and Welfare, Audit Agency—Region III, "Review of Nursing Care Provided by Nursing Homes in Maryland," Audit Control No. 50151-03, May 8, 1975, p. 3. Mimeographed; Minnesota Report, p. 4; Oregon Report, p. 3; U.S., Department of Health, Education, and Welfare, Audit Agency—Region I, "Review of Selected Aspects of Skilled Nursing Facility and Intermediate Care Facility Level of Care Operations Under Title XIX of the Social Security Act, As Administered by the State of Rhode Island," Audit Control No. 50166-01, May 16, 1975, pp. 6–8. Mimeographed; U.S., Department of Health, Education, and Welfare, Audit Agency—Region VIII, "Report on Review of Level of Care in Nursing Facilities Under Title XIX of the Social Security Act, State of Utah," Audit Control No. 08-50151, January 22, 1975, pp. 1–2. Mimeographed; U.S., Department of Health, Education, and Welfare, Audit Agency—Region III, "Controls Established by State Health Department (Virginia) Over Nursing Care Provided to Eligible Medicaid Patients," Audit Control No. 50150-03, September 25, 1974, pp. 4–8. Mimeographed; and U.S., Department of Health, Education, and Welfare, Audit Agency—Region III, "Review of Management Controls and Operating Practices For Level of Care Provided Medicaid Recipients in Nursing Homes, West Virginia Department of Welfare," Audit Control No. 50152-03, December, 1974, p. 2. Mimeographed.

51. U.S., Congress, Senate, Special Committee on Aging, Subcommittee on Long-Term Care, *The Litany of Nursing Home Abuses And An Examination of the Roots of Controversy*, Supporting Paper No. 1 (Washington, D.C.: Government Printing Office, 1974), pp. 173–80, 183–85.

52. Indiana Report, p. 15; Maryland Report, p. 5; and Rhode Island Report, p. 15.

53. Indiana Report, p. 11; and New York State Moreland Act Commission on Nursing Homes and Residential Facilities, *Regulating Nursing Home Care: The Paper Tigers* (New York: New York State Moreland Act Commission, 1975), p. 3.

54. New York State Moreland Act Commission, *Regulating Nursing Home Care*, p. 3; U.S., Congress, Senate, Special Committee on Aging, *Litany of Abuses*, pp. 169–73, 180–82, 188–93, 196–99; Maine Report, p. 22; Oregon Report, pp. 17–18; Rhode Island Report, p. 16; West Virginia Report, pp. 4–5; and U.S., Department of Health, Education, and Welfare, Audit Agency—Region III, "Report on Practices and Procedures Relating to Income and Assets of Medicaid Recipients in State and Private Nursing Homes in the District of Columbia," Audit Control No. 50164-03, June 13, 1975, pp. 4–5. Mimeographed.

55. U.S., Congress, Senate, Special Committee on Aging, *Litany of Abuses*, pp. 205–8.

56. U.S., Congress, Senate, Special Committee on Aging, *Nursing Home Care*, pp. 45–53, 66.

57. U.S., Congress, Senate, Special Committee on Aging, *Nursing Home Care*, p. 79.

58. Interview with Dr. George Warner, Special Assistant (for long-term care) to the Deputy Commissioner of Health, State of New York, January 7, 1976.

59. Ellen W. Jones, *Patient Classification for Long-Term Care: User's Manual*, DHEW Publication No. (HRA) 74-3107 (Washington, D.C.: Government Printing Office, 1974).

60. U.S., Department of Health, Education, and Welfare, Office of Nursing Home Affairs, *Long-Term Care Facility Improvement Study*, Introductory Report, DHEW Publication No. (OS) 76-50021 (Washington, D.C.: Government Printing Office, 1975).

61. New York State Moreland Act Commission, *Regulating Nursing Home Care*, p. 29. The New York State Health Department is currently in the process of developing a detailed facility evaluation and rating system which provides specific guidance to inspectors for evaluating whether compliance with requirements in eight basic areas—nursing, dietary, activities, environment, physician care, rehabilitation therapy, social services, and physical plant—is superior, very good, good, poor, or unacceptable. Facilities will then be rated on an A to F scale based on the number of superior, very good, etc., ratings.

62. Massachusetts Report, p. 10.

63. U.S., Congress, Senate, Special Committee on Aging, *Nursing Home Care*, p. 79.

64. Minnesota Report, p. 39; Maryland Report, p. 2; Illinois Report, p. 7; Indiana Report, p. 8; Massachusetts Report, p. 2; Rhode Island Report, pp. 9–10; New York State Moreland Act Commission, *Regulating Nursing Home Care*, pp. 10, 21–22, 62; and "Major Reforms Proposed for State Medicaid Program," *New York Times*, October 14, 1975, p. 41. (New Jersey edition.)

65. Maine Report, p. 10; and "Nursing Homes Show Progress," *New York Times*, January 12, 1976, p. 32.

66. Amitai Etzioni, "Nursing Homes: New Rules Are Not Enough," *Medical Care Review* 32, no. 7 (1975), p. 819; and Wilson, "The Dead Hand," p. 41.

67. U.S., Congress, Senate, Special Committee on Aging, *Nursing Home Care*, p. 82.

68. New York State Moreland Act Commission, *Regulating Nursing Home Care*, pp. 69–83; and Wilson, "The Dead Hand," p. 41.

69. U.S., Congress, Senate, Special Committee on Aging, *Nursing Home Care*, p. 84.

70. Mary A. Mendelson, *Tender Loving Greed* (New York: Knopf, 1974), pp. 219–20.

71. "Moreland Nursing Home Report Cites Rockefeller," *New York Times*, February 26, 1976, pp. 1, 61.

72. "Battles are Shaping Up Over Nursing Homes as Operators Threaten to Refuse Added Patients," *New York Times*, November 12, 1975, p. 40.

73. "Enforcing Nursing-Home Convictions," *New York Times*, February 5, 1976, p. 60.

74. U.S., Congress, Senate, Special Committee on Aging, *Nursing Home Care*, p. 80.

75. Cohen, *Long-Term Care*, p. 12.

76. Illinois Report, p. 31; Indiana Report, pp. 4, 6; Massachusetts Report, p. 2; Minnesota Report, pp. 5, 23–24; Oregon Report, p. 11; Rhode Island Report, p. 4; Utah Report, pp. 5–7.

77. New York State Moreland Act Commissin, *Regulating Nursing Home Care*, pp. 46, 59.

78. See Ruchlin et al., "The Long-Term Care Marketplace"; and Robert L. Kane et al., "Caution: Nursing Homes May Be Hazardous To Your Health," Department of Family and Community Medicine, University of Utah College of Medicine, 1976. Mimeographed.

79. New York State Moreland Act Commission, *Regulating Nursing Home Care*, p. 9; Maryland Report, p. 11; Kentucky Report, pp. 5, 8; and New Hampshire Report, pp. 3–4.

80. R. Hopkins Holmberg and Nancy N. Anderson, "Implications of Ownership for Nursing Home Care," *Medical Care*, VI, No. 4 (1968), 300–7; Samuel Levey et al., "An

Appraisal of Nursing Home Care," *Journal of Gerontology* 28, no. 2 (1973), pp. 222–28; and New York State Moreland Act Commission on Nursing Homes and Residential Facilities, *Reimbursement of Nursing Home Property Costs: Pruning the Money Tree* (New York: New York State Moreland Act Commission on Nursing Homes and Residential Facilities, 1976), pp. 5, 120–22.

81. For a summary of some of the arguments advanced in support of a public utility approach see Lehamae McCoy, "The Nursing Home As A Public Utility," *Journal of Economic Issues* 5, no. 1 (1971), pp. 67–76.

82. William C. Thomas, *Nursing Homes and Public Policy: Drift and Decision in New York State* (Ithaca: Cornell University Press, 1969), Chapters 3–5.

83. The detailed reimbursement proposal is described in Hirsch Ruchlin et al., "An Incentive Reimbursement Proposal for Financing Long-Term Care Services," Contract No. HEW-OS-74-176, and summarized in Ruchlin et al., "The Long-Term Care Marketplace," pp. 982–86. For a similar and independently developed proposal see Amitai Etzioni et al., "Public Management of Health and Home Care for the Aged and Disabled.. (New York: Center for Policy Research, 1975). Mimeographed.

84. For a detailed exposition of how this process works and for the high after tax profits (approximately 20 percent) that can be reaped under it, see New York State Moreland Act Commission, *Reimbursement of Nursing Home Property Costs*, Chs. 3–4.

85. Green and Nader, pp. 888–89.

86. Jane L. Barney, "Community Presence As A Key to Quality of Life in Nursing Homes," *American Journal of Public Health* 64, no. 3 (1974), p. 267.

87. For a discussion of types of taxes used by federal/state/local governments to raise revenue, and the effectiveness of each type of tax in ensuring a suitable match between responsbility for providing services and access to tax revenue, see Hirsch S. Ruchlin and Daniel C. Rogers, *Economics and Health Care* (Springfield, Ill.: Charles C. Thomas Publishers, 1973), pp. 231–45.

88. Thomas, *Nursing Homes*, chs. 2–5.

89. Barney, "Community Presence," p. 265; Etzioni, "Nursing Homes: New Rules Are Not Enough," p. 820; Judith W. LaVor, "Intermediate Care Facilities: Expectations vs. Reality," Disability Long Term Care Study, OASPE, August 1974, p. 12. Mimeographed; and Herbert Shore, "Long-Term Care Regulations: Counterproductive and Costly," *Hospitals* 49, no. 20 (1975), pp. 57–61.

90. Shore, "Long-Term Care," p. 59.

91. Rush-Presbyterian-St. Luke's Medical Center, *A Methodology For the Evaluation of Quality of Life and Care in Long-Term Care Facilities*, Contract No. HSM 110-72-400, Document No. PB 236-725 (Springfield, Va.: National Technical Information Service, 1974).

92. Robert H. Brook, *Quality of Care Assessment: A Comparison of Five Methods of Peer Review*, DHEW Publication No. HRA-74-3100 (Washington, D.C.: Government Printing Office, 1973).

93. One exception is the State of Illinois where such a system has been developed and implemented since 1973. For a discussion of this system see Donald B. St. John et al., "An Automated System for the Regulation and Medical Review of Long-Term Care Facilities and Patients," *American Journal of Public Health* 63, no. 6 (1973), pp. 619–30.

94. Rashi Fein, "On Achieving Access and Equity in Health Care," *Milbank Memorial Fund Quarterly* 50, no. 4, Part II (1972), p. 175.

5
THE AUDITING OF LONG-TERM CARE AND DISABILITY PROGRAMS

Robert M. Dias

CURRENT AUDITING PROCEDURES

Introduction

The spiraling of costs and the increasing allocation of resources in the long-term care and disability fields have concentrated much attention, both governmental and nongovernmental, on the question of whether or not long-term care disability programs are being adequately audited. There have been many publicized instances of inadequate care, misuse of funds, fraud, excessive expenditures for administration, and widespread Medicare and Medicaid abuses. Some of the information has come from the news media and other private sources, but a great deal has originated from the audit activities of the federal and state government. For the most part, however, program officials and administrators have shown only a passing interest in the audit function. Legislators and policymakers, for example, have been inclined to view auditing as a technically oriented function concerned with after-the-fact fiscal disclosure. But recent publicity surrounding programs in the field has given rise to a new interest in auditing and has helped to raise some important questions.

The first question concerns the scope of government audit. Obviously, the monitoring of the fiscal aspects of a program's operation is an important and necessary part of an audit. But should the auditing team look further and evaluate the effectiveness and efficiency of a program? Should it, in other words, look beyond the balance sheet and into the program's management and objectives? A second issue centers on the selection of an appropriate group to perform the auditing. A decision has to be made concerning which agency, at what level of government, is to be responsible for the audit. In addition, consideration must be given to the disciplines that are to be represented on an auditing team and the method by which the audit is financed. Finally, the desired end result of an audit must be clearly defined so that recommendations can be made and their implementation enforced.

This chapter analyzes these and other pertinent questions relating to the audit of long-term care and disability programs. Conclusions are drawn insofar as evidence and experience permit. The chapter remains, however, only a guide; it is intended to generate discussion and to provide directions for further investigation. The broad scope of the paper means that it cannot be a substitute for an agency's critical analysis of its own strengths and weaknesses, but it should provide a foundation upon which agencies can build more comprehensive and productive auditing procedures.

An Overview of Current Procedures

The audit work that is done in the field of long-term care and disability is conducted by the Health, Education, and Welfare Audit Agency, the U.S. General Accounting Office and state auditors. The latter also employ CPA's and private consultants. The following is a brief description of each of these auditing agents.

HEW Audit Agency (HEWAA):

This agency, established in 1965 in the Office of the Assistant Secretary Comptroller, has a staff of about 900 professionals located in ten regional offices, 40 branch offices, and a headquarters. The agency has as its charter the responsibility for conducting comprehensive audits of all department programs, functions, and activities. Its objectives are twofold: (1) to determine whether the department's operations are being conducted economically and efficiently, and (2) to provide a reasonable degree of assurance that funds are expended properly and for the purpose for which they were intended.[1] HEW operates about 375 programs budgeted at $130 billion.

U.S. General Accounting Office (GAO):

The U.S. General Accounting Office is an independent, nonpolitical agency in the legislative branch of the government. It provides the Congress, its committees, and members with information, analyses, and recommendations concerning operations of the government, primarily those of the executive branch. GAO's concern is that federal departments and agencies, through their programs and activities, carry out the mandate or intent of legislation enacted by Congress. The GAO professional staff numbers about 3,300.

State Auditors

The size and capability of state audit groups vary greatly. They also differ significantly in terms of the scope of work they undertake and the extent of their authority. Most of the work performed is fiscal and compliance-oriented. The bulk of local government auditing in this country is performed by certified public accountants. Many states also contract with private firms for special studies and evaluations in specific areas. Some of the analyses made by these consultants are similar to the type of analytical work performed in a management or performance audit.

The audit universe for which the three auditing groups are responsible is, in terms of the number of entities and their dollar cost, very large. Table 5.1 gives an approximate picture of the magnitude of the auditing responsibility.

With some understanding of the groups that perform audits in the long-term and disability fields, we can take up the question of what constitutes an audit. The guidelines that the HEW Audit Agency follow in reviewing department programs provide some insight into the way in which the audit function is interpreted at the present time. As part of an executive department of the federal government, the HEW Audit Agency is subject to audit policy guidance from the Office of Management and Budget.[2] Audits are defined in the guidelines as systematic reviews or appraisals to determine whether: (1) financial operations are properly conducted and financial reports are presented fairly; (2) applicable laws and regulations have been complied with; (3) resources are managed and used in an economical and efficient manner; and (4) desired results and objectives are being achieved in an effective manner. In addition, for those agencies that administer grant-in-aid programs through state and local governments, a financial compliance audit should be conducted at least once every two years. Every audit may cover one or more of the aspects listed above each time and is to be conducted under general standards promulgated by the GAO.

The Standards for Audit of Governmental Organizations, Programs, Activities, and Functions (known as the "Yellow Book"), published by the Comptroller General in 1972, specified that an audit of a governmental program, function, or activity should encompass: (1) an examination of *financial transactions*, accounts, and reports, including an evaluation of

TABLE 5.1

The Audit Universe

Area	Number of Audit Entities
Medicaid:	
State Agencies	54
Insurance Companies	—*
Hospitals	—
Skilled Nursing Homes	20,000
Medicare:	
Intermediaries	137
Direct Dealers	350
State Agencies	54
Providers	10,450
Rehabilitation Services:	
Vocational Rehabilitation	54
Other	54
Older Americans Act	54
State, Section 1864	54
States, Disability Determination	54
Professional Service Review Organizations	120
Health Maintenance Organizations	180

*Major audit areas for which statistics are not available.

Source: U.S. Department of HEW, HEW Audit Agency, Annual Work Plan, FY 1976, p. 6.

compliance aspects; (2) a review of *efficiency and economy* in the use of resources; and (3) a review to determine whether desired *program results* are *effectively achieved.*

Financial and compliance audit seeks to determine whether financial operations are properly conducted, whether the financial reports of an audited entity are presented fairly, and whether the entity has complied with applicable laws and regulations.

Reviews for efficiency and economy ask whether the organization is getting the most it can for the money and other resources it spends or consumes. The auditor is concerned with the way the management of an entity has chosen to organize and operate. For example, in such a review it is not sufficient to know that a service that was purchased was received and paid for at the billed price; the auditor must also consider whether the service was needed, whether it was actually used productively, and whether it could have been obtained at a lower price.

Reviewing and reporting on program results, or effectiveness, is on the leading edge of what has to be done in auditing. The nature of an effectiveness audit can be seen more clearly by contrasting it with audits of other types already discussed. Thus, in audits for compliance, efficiency, or economy, the things an entity has chosen to do are measured more or less as if they were ends in themselves. In effectiveness auditing, those same things that the entity has chosen to do are weighed in a different balance. The question to be asked is this: Has the entity chosen to do the right things in order to achieve its goals? To assess effectiveness, an auditor must know what goals have been established for or by an antity and must be able to measure the results.

The standards specified by the Comptroller General place on officials who authorize and prescribe the scope of governmental audits the responsibility to provide audit work broad enough to fulfill the need of all potential users of the results of such audits. The standards are not intended to prevent such officials from authorizing specific assignments or from authorizing special audits, nor are they intended to prevent auditors from performing such audits. However, those responsible for authorizing government audits are charged with the knowledge that, for most government programs, their full responsibility for obtaining audit work is not discharged unless the full scope of audit work set forth in the standard is performed.

The Yellow Book sets federal standards that provide for broad-scope auditing. These standards are intended to be applicable at *all* levels of government, and are applicable whether audits are performed by federal, state, or local government auditors, by independent public accountants, or by others.

Audit standards are also published by the American Institute of Certified Public Accountants (AICPA). The AICPA standards are directed primarily toward audits made with the objective of expressing *opinions on whether the financial statements* of an organization fairly present its operations and financial position. They are *not* directed toward the broad management concerns addressed by the GAO standards. In the past, the public accounting profession has been opposed to the idea of expanding audit processes to include management and efficiency reviews and performance and effectiveness reviews. It has tended to argue that these forms of review should be performed by the internal audit staffs of the organizations themselves. More recently, however, some substantial changes have taken place at the policy level of the AICPA. The climate now seems ripe for the universal implementation of the federal standards to all audits in the public sector. Nevertheless, while the profession has expressed some willingness to undertake reviews of program efficiency and results, it has tended to regard such operations as *management advising services* rather than parts of the *audit function* proper. Most public accountants, in their public sector audits, do not include a review of compliance as a part of the financial examination. Whether or not the GAO audit standards are accepted at the working level is a crucial issue in determining the nature and subsequent impact of audits.

Present federal regulations and guidelines relating to long-term care and disability programs are vague as to the intent and arrangements for audit, and very few give specific details as to what compliance program elements the auditor should examine. This lack of clarity sets the long-term care programs apart from other public programs, notably those directed by the Community Services Administration (CSA), the former Office of Economic Opportunity. In the case of the CSA programs, fairly specific guides for audit are contained within the authorizing legislation or have been administratively developed. Part of the current problem in the long-term care and disability field is that program managers continue to believe that auditors are too absorbed in accounting and fiscal technicalities to successfully conduct audits of performance and program effectiveness that could produce information of real value to managers and administrators. There are also some managers who still doubt whether auditors are qualified to evaluate program management practices and procedures. These managers regard fiscal review as the sole domain of the accountant and program or performance reviews as the exclusive domain of the administrator. The resolution of this issue will depend on continued communication between auditors and managers and may demonstrate that audit is a useful management tool.

Department of Health, Education, and Welfare Audit Agency

The HEWAA oprations are tied to its annual work plan. During preparation of the plan, input is requested from operating agencies as well as department officials. The work plan details the areas to be reviewed, the number of audit sites to be included in each review, and the amount of resources allocated to do the job. The factors used by the audit agency to determine the entities and programs to be reviewed include:

1. the sensitivity of the area in terms of congressional and departmental interest;
2. requests from department officials;
3. the amount of federal funds involved;
4. prior audit experiences and the time of last audit; and
5. statutory or other mandated audit coverage.[3]

TABLE 5.2

HEWAA Resource Allocation

Programs	Planned Man-Years of Effort FY 1975	FY 1976
Medicaid	50.5	76.7
Medicare	66.2	53.2
Disability Determination Program	7.2	9.5
Vocational Rehabilitation	7.0	10.0
Developmental Disability	0	2.0
Administration on Aging	16.6	23.0
HMO Program	23.0	4.0
PSROs	1.0	5.0
SSI Program	7.3*	140.4
Total	242.8	323.8
Total HEWAA Resources	1,094.0	860.0

*Over 102 man-years were actually expended in this area.

Source: U.S. Department of HEW, HEW Audit Agency, Annual Work Plans for FY 1975 and FY 1976, summary of various pages therein.

Areas having nationwide impact are usually programmed by the audit agency's headquarters divisions. Various regional audit staffs furnish work-plan input regarding regional requests and problems.

Table 5.2 is a summary of HEWAA staff resources allocated to long-term care and disability programs and shows the relatively limited resources available to the Department for monitoring the various programs.

Most long-term care and disability audits conducted by the agency are based on an audit guide prepared by the headquarters division. In some cases, the audit guides are prepared by a regional office. For the most part, the agency's current audit posture leans toward questions of program compliance as well as economy of operations, and where appropriate, effectiveness in accomplishment of program goals. When the results of audit indicate the possibility of fraud, the agency coordinates its activities with the department's Office of Investigations and Security. The results of audit are formally communicated to the appropriate officials via an audit report. The agency is also responsible for evaluating the adequacy of audits

TABLE 5.3

HEWAA Scheduled Audits

| | Number of Audits | |
Programs	FY 1975	FY 1976
Medicaid	49	110
Medicare	120	85
Disability Determination Program	19	21
Vocational Rehabilitation	12	16
Developmental Disabilities	0	2
Administration on Aging	14	21
HMOs	54	23
PSROs	1	9
SSI Program	139	113
TOTAL	408	401

Source: U.S. Department of HEW, HEW Audit Agency, Annual Work Plans for FY 1975 and FY 1976, summary of various pages therein.

made by certified public accountants of provider costs under the Medicare program.

Table 5.3 shows the number of audits scheduled to be conducted under the FY 1975 and FY 1976 work plans.

From a cross-section of the long-term care and disability reports issued by the HEWAA between July 1, 1973, and June 30, 1975, the following general areas consistently produced the most problems: 1) Lack of adequate program controls, monitoring, and follow-up action to ensure that department and state regulations are met. Deficiencies of this nature were consistently found in audits pertaining to such areas as utilization review, medical team activity, and nursing home certification; 2) Poor financial management. This finding includes such items as inadequate cost controls, excessive reimbursement, and duplicate payments; 3) Failure to provide services to recipients in a timely manner; and 4) Lack of coordination between various long-term care and disability programs.

Two good examples of the type of areas audited by HEWAA and the types of recommendations made in an audit report are provided by a closer look at the Medicare and Medicaid audits made over the 24-month period mentioned above. The audit agency performs audits at 53 state agencies and 129 intermediaries and contract carriers that participate in Medicare. State agencies survey hospitals and other health facilities and certify their compliance with Medicare conditions of participation. Contractors process and pay claims for the health services provided to Medicare beneficiaries. In FY 1975 the contractors made Medicare benefit payments totaling $13.8 billion. Briefly, the areas audited are:

1. *Administrative Costs*: Audit determines whether the required reports of reimbursable costs submitted to SSA present fairly the allowable costs of administration; it also evaluates the adequacy of state/contractor accounting systems and internal controls. In FY 1975 the states and contractors incurred costs of $430 million in Medicare administration.

2. *Provider Certifications*: Audit at the state agency level looks into the effectiveness of procedures for assuring that providers are adequately surveyed and resurveyed at the appropriate time. They also review those procedures that indicate whether or not providers meet the standards for participation.

3. *Claims Processing Systems*: Audit examines the adequacy and efficiency of intermediary and carrier systems for processing Medicare claims. Tests are made of processing operations and of the controls in effect to prevent such abuses as duplicate payments, overpayments, and excessive utilization of hospital and medical services.

4. *Provider Reimbursement*: Audits of intermediaries test the propriety of audits and settlements of cost reports submitted annually by providers of service. Audit tests have focused on related organization transactions, owners' compensation, and administration salaries that are problem areas in proprietary facilities. For carriers, tests are made of the reasonable charges reimbursed to physicians and of the utilization profiles established by carriers to detect patterns of excessive physicians' services.

During FY 1974 and 1975 the audit agency issued 187 audit reports covering Medicare administrative costs of about $573 million. The reports recommended adjustment of unallowable costs totaling about $9 million. Many of the reports also identified the following weaknesses in auditee financial management and offered recommendations for improvement in these areas.

1. Inadequate state surveys and follow-ups on deficiencies at health facilities, resulting in the certification of providers not in compliance with all Medicare conditions of participation.

2. Duplicate payments for physicians' services due to inadequate contractor procedures for detecting duplicative Medicare claims submitted by providers and beneficiaries.

3. Unnecessary coinsurance payments by beneficiaries for preadmission hospital outpatient services that should have been processed as inpatient services. Beneficiaries must pay 20 percent of the charges for hospital outpatient services.

4. Improperly set parameters for detecting overutilization of health services and inadequate medical reviews of suspected overutilization cases.

5. Unrecovered overpayments to providers caused by lax collection procedures by the contractors.

The Medicaid program is designed to help finance states' plans for providing medical assistance to their low-income population. The federal government shares the cost of both direct and administrative expenses with participating states. The Social and Rehabilitation Service (SRS) provides federal guidance and overall regulatory control, while states determine client eligibility and make payments to doctors, dentists, druggists, nursing homes, hospitals, and other vendors providing medical services. The areas audited are: a) eligibility—audits focus on recipients for federal assistance and the accuracy of claims paid to vendors providing medical services to them; b) nursing home administration—audits cover the level of care, required medical reviews, control over patient personal assets, compliance with safety codes and reimbursement procedures; c) pharmaceuticals—audits examine the possible overutilization of drugs, the adequacy of state drug formularies and pricing methods; and d) administrative charges—audits focus on the reliability of overhead cost representations.

In 1969 the audit agency submitted to the secretary a summary of principal problems noted in audits of 16 selected states. The areas of most concern centered on: (1) duplicate payments, excessive rates and fees, and other types of erroneous charges; (2) the lack of systematic reviews of the utilization of services; and (3) the need for improved procedures in determining eligibility and operating quality control programs. The nature and extent of the agency's subsequent findings indicated a continuing trend of weaknesses in the same areas which, if not corrected, would seriously detract from program performance. The agency identified the following areas in need of improvement: the procedures for determining and rechecking client eligibility; the propriety and timeliness of vendor claims and controls over improper payments; nursing home compliance with life/safety code requirements and the level of care provided patients; the reliability of drug pricing and prescribed use for patients; and the accuracy of state claims for reimbursable administrative charges.[4]

This brief summary of the auditing of two long-term care and disability programs points up a major problem: Program deficiencies recur even after they have been identified by audit reports. When considering the marginal record of the department and the states in taking action on audit recommendations, it is not difficult to understand the fiscal crisis and abuses in long-term care and disability progrms. If *known problems* identified by audit cannot be resolved quickly and effectively, there can be no point in going into more sophisticated and controversial programmatic audits.

Very few of the audit reports reviewed for this study made reference to the overall adequacy of internal control. On the other hand, many of the reports reviewed contained the formula, "We have recommended that controls be established to . . . ." These recommendations are usually directed at improving internal controls that pertain to specific functional areas. The problem here is that adequate internal control over financial, administrative, and management transactions is absolutely necessary for successful program operations. The serious nature, magnitude, and recurrence of many of the HEWAA findings indicate that there are major deficiencies in overall long-term care and disability program internal control systems and procedures at all levels that have not been resolved. Instead of merely recommending that internal control be improved, the audit agency might take the initiative to provide specific requirements and guidelines for establishing controls.

U.S. General Accounting Office

The GAO conducts reviews of various HEW long-term care and disability programs on an ongoing basis. Resident GAO staffs are located at all of the department's agencies in the Washington metropolitan area and Baltimore. Field work is conducted by staffs located at various regional and branch offices nationwide. Technically, GAO reports related to long-term care and disability programs fall into two categories: those studies of specific programs in specific states that are requested by Congress, and national studies that usually cover selected program activities in six or eight states.

Not unlike the audit reports issued by the HEWAA, the GAO reports provide a valuable flow of information on fiscal and compliance activities, and in some cases, on the effectiveness of the Medicare and Medicaid programs and the efficiency of operations. Unfortunately, the data contained in the GAO reports have not been fully utilized by the department, and many recommendations have not been implemented. Other recommendations have only been partially implemented and, with the exception of the HEWAA, the data have not been used to trigger or supplement the department's own long-term care and disability research and evaluation efforts.

The GAO audit reports consistently pinpoint deficiencies in department planning, coordination, internal control, fiscal management, program management, and compliance activities. These deficiencies have been found at all levels—federal, state, and local and involved various department entities, state agencies, intermediaries, hospitals, and nursing homes. In addition, an inordinately large number of the reports contain audit findings that pertain to HEW program regulations. GAO has continually criticized the department for: (1) tardiness in developing vital program regulations; (2) use of inadequate regulations; and (3) failure to enforce regulations.[5]

The following list of GAO projects provides some idea of the approach taken by a GAO audit team and the nature of their findings. This list is, of course, only a partial look at GAO audit activities. In general, reports are issued which cover: Medicaid fraud and abuse; hospital compliance with Medicaid reimbursement regulations; deficiencies in rate-setting procedures; eligibility requirements; Early and Periodic Screening, Diagnosis and Treatment Program (EPSDT) implementation; control requirements for HMOs; service cutbacks in home health care; problems of outpatient care; and comparisons of federal and private fiscal intermediaries. The projects described below were underway as of February 1976.

Survey of State Utilization Review Programs for Noninstitutional Services under Medicaid: This survey is designed to obtain specific information on the various states' systems used to detect and prevent overutilization, underutilization, and inappropriate utilization of medical services provided by physicians, laboratories, and other noninstitutional providers.

Review of Management of Medicaid Patients' Personal Funds by Nursing Homes: This review is being made in five states. So far GAO identified widespread abuse and mismanagement of the personal funds maintained by facilities on behalf of patients.

Review of Medicaid Insuring Agreements: A Medicaid insuring agreement is a contract between a state and a private firm under which the contractor agrees to pay all eligible claims for the services covered by the contract in return for a fixed capitation payment. Two of the objectives of this review are to determine: (a) whether appropriate procedures were followed in the awards of such contracts, and (b) if the insuring agreements have actually produced the intended cost controls and program savings.

Review of Recoveries from Liable Third Parties for Health Services Covered by Medicaid: This review involves an evaluation of state systems to avoid or recover the costs of health services provided to Medicaid recipients that third parties such as private health insurance companies are responsible for paying.

Review of Nursing Home Costs Under Medicaid: This review is being made in four states. It is designed to identify the extent to which skilled nursing facilities overstate costs or make claims for expenses not covered under Medicaid in order to receive additional reimbursement.

Review of the Social Security Administration's Medicare Program Integrity Function: This review focuses on an evaluation of the scope and adequacy of the Social Security Administration's investigations of fraud and abuse in Medicare. Coordination with Medicaid investigators and the extent of state Medicare investigations were also covered. To date, GAO has found that: a) Medicare program integrity activity was mostly oriented toward answering beneficiary complaints about physicians' services. Self-initiated investigations and investigations of institutional providers were limited; b) many of the investigations were not adequate and cases were closed when further investigations appeared to be warranted; c) at times Medicare carriers conducted investigations that exceeded the scope of their authority. These investigations were often inadequate.

Review of Controls over the Quality and Costs of Laboratory Services under Four Federally Funded Health Programs: The main finding of this review so far is that physicians are obtaining tests from independent laboratories and then billing as if they had performed the tests themselves. The physicians add large markups to the amounts the laboratories charged. This technique works because the charge allowed a physician is higher than the charge allowed an independent laboratory for the same test. GAO also indicated a lack of control over the quality of laboratory services. For example GAO found that some carriers are not checking to make sure that the laboratories are certified before paying them; carriers are not aware, or act as if they were not aware, that many tests billed by physicians are in fact performed by independent laboratories.[6]

State Auditors

In every state, there is at least one central audit or "post audit" organization headed by an elected or appointed auditor. A central audit department is authorized to conduct audits of state operations, including most programs funded with federal grants. Such audit functions report to the governor, the legislature, and/or the electorate rather than state program administrators. By law, or by practice, state audit reports are public documents in all 50 states.

At the state level there are also state internal program-level auditors who perform program audits of federally assisted programs and state operations. In most cases they report to the program manager and operate independently of any state central audit department. Their internal reports are often not released to the public.

State auditing is significantly dissimilar in purpose, use, and form from the so-called independent audit by certified public accountants. State auditing is a political function and its purpose is to serve as a means of achieving public accountability for government action. The state audit function is useful to the extent to which it achieves such accountability. Over the past several years, the state audit function in some states has been expanded so as to provide public accounting of an increased range of governmental activities and to give increasingly specific recognition to the functional interrelationships between the audit and legislative functions.

TABLE 5.4

New York State Audit Resources

Agency	Number of People
Office of the State Comptroller	300
Office of Welfare Inspector General	100
Department of Social Services	460
Deputy Attorney General for Health and Social Service	210
Department of Health	135
Commissioner of Investigations	40
TOTAL	1,245

Source: New York State FY 1976 Legislative Budget Summary, p. 132.

One way of gauging the capabilities of state auditing is to look at the resources available in a particular state. New York provides a good example. In New York State there are six major audit and investigatory groups which, in varying degrees, oversee the propriety of expenditure of federal funds. Collectively, these agencies employ about 1,245 people. Table 5.4 shows the breakdown by agency. These various agencies perform audits and conduct investigations of state and local programs, including those programs emanating from federal sources, including HEW. In New York State, HEW spends about $12 billion annually, of which the Medicaid and Public Assistance programs account for about one-fourth, or $3 billion. It should also be noted that New York City employs about 750 auditors and investigators. The staffs of the various New York State audit groups consist of accountants, attorneys, and investigators. Salaries range from $10,000 to $40,000 per year. It is obvious from this example that there is a substantial audit capability at the state and local levels.

The application and continuing development of new forms of state auditing demonstrates that the state audit function can be used to attain additional control and accountability over long-term care and disability programs. Recent developments in regard to the program review aspects of state auditing contribute to an expanding awareness of the potential of the state audit function. State audit is the subject of growing attention, particularly among legislators and professional accounting groups at the state level. However, there is no certainty that this development will lead to the wider employment of state audits. Nor is it certain that where employed they will be used effectively. Indeed, there are several factors which seem to weigh against such widened, effective, and sustained use of the state audit function. In the first place, there must be legislative acceptance of the need for additional control of long-term care and disability program administration, which may depend more heavily upon the "politics of accountability" than upon whatever objective evidence may be brought before a state legislature. Secondly, it is necessary that the state audit function be viewed as a potential means by which input regarding the effectiveness and economy of operations can be obtained. Recent developments in several states demonstrate that state audit entities can provide such input. This conclusion, however, is opposed to the prevailing tendency to equate the state audit function with the conduct of financial review. There is no inherent reason why state audit efforts should be employed only to measure the financial aspects of government administration. Nevertheless, the conduct of fiscal-compliance auditing is widely viewed as being an end in itself. State audit is seldom viewed as an instrument of public accountability for the full scope of management and financial activities related to program operations and effectiveness.

The effective use of state audit resources requires: (a) the existence of a mutually responsive working relationship between state and federal audit groups, and (b) proper employment of the analytic and subject skills required to conduct meaningful examination of government operations, management, programs, and policies. Neither of these conditions is readily achieved or easily maintained. A viable and mutually responsive working relationship between state and federal auditors on long-term care and disability programs can be realized only through visible departmental commitment to the concept. This relationship is continually subject to the many and conflicting pressures arising from the politics of accountability. To acquire and maintain the analytic and subject competence required to conduct expanded forms of audit may be so costly as to inhibit employment of these audit methods. Even in the case of operational and management auditing, where the requisite skills are relatively well defined, recruitment of qualified personnel may prove difficult, and the retraining of existing staff is likely to be both time-consuming and costly.

Finally, a decision to expand the scope and intensity of state audit programs is not necessarily permanent. Such action is likely to engender continuing controversy, including efforts to redefine and limit the scope of public audit. The use of operational and program audit is likely to alter the distribution of information required to control governmental actions. Such an effect is likely to be opposed by persons or groups who believe they influence or control state government administration, and who view the existing norm of public accounting as best serving their interests. An expanded role for state auditors requires the resolution of some long-standing objections or problems raised by department and state officials. Briefly, these objections can be summarized as follows.

1. States are not qualified to conduct acceptable audits.

2. Where state auditors are appointed, the audit results are subject to excessive political bias.

3. A state's interest in the management and effectiveness of programs does not coincide in many cases with federal objectives; therefore, federal auditors are necessary to maintain control.

4. State audit functions vary from state to state. Some state auditors authority is restricted, whereas others have wide responsibility, even down to the local level, to audit every government dollar that flows into the state.

5. States resist performing audits for federal use unless they are adequately reimbursed.

6. Federal program managers resist complying with Federal Management Circular 74-4, which established the guidelines for reimbursing state governments for administrative (including audit) costs incurred in operating federal grant programs.

7. Program managers at the state and federal level resist efforts to increase state-performed audits.

8. In several instances, provisions for paying for audit work have been written into program regulations. However, the money is diverted from states' central audit offices.

9. Management of the executive branch needs strengthening where it concerns the enforcement of directives and circulars that bear on the problem of state audits and reimbursement.

10. Federal departments are so large and perform such diverse services that they are difficult to manage. The same is frequently true of state governments. Elected and appointed officials have difficulty influencing or modifying the close relationships that develop between state program managers and their federal counterparts. Federal and state program managers as a consequence often act autonomously and can successfully ignore audit directives and efforts aimed at simplifying procedures and streamlining operations.

Some of the more important of these issues are taken up in the following section on *Auditing Problems and Recommendations*.

Summary

The auditing of long-term care and disability programs is the responsibility of three separate groups: the HEWAA, the GAO, and state auditors. The first two are federal agencies that conduct wide-ranging audits covering program compliance as well as fiscal practices. The adverse publicity that some long-term care and disability programs have recently been receiving does not, on close examination of past audit reports, reveal many deficiencies not already identified in audit reports. The conclusion to be drawn is that the findings and recommendations of auditing teams are not having a sufficient impact on administrators and managers, and, as a consequence, program performances are not being improved in the areas indicated by audit.

State audits are primarily fiscally oriented, but there is a growing awareness that their capabilities and their subsequent impact on program performance could be much greater. The redefining of the audit function and the shifting of the burden to a more local level are the cornerstones for reforming current auditing procedures. These policy initiatives are discussed in the next section.

AUDITING PROBLEMS AND RECOMMENDATIONS: INTRODUCTION

Certain characteristics of the auditing procedures described in the first section of this chapter have given rise to financial and operational problems. First, the amount of resources allocated to the audit function is fairly limited, and long-term care and disability programs are growing at a faster rate than audit capabilities. Although a simple solution would be to allocate more funds for auditing, it is not clear that this would be the most efficient solution, given the existing structure of the audit program. At present there seems to be a duplication of the auditing effort by different agencies at different levels of government. Elimination of this duplication through reorganization and coordination would not only improve the overall efficiency of auditing but also release resources that could then be applied to the monitoring of an increased number of entitites. If federal and state audit teams are to coordinate their auditing efforts, however, certain complications should be anticipated; reorganization might lead to a number of subsidiary problems such as highly complex reimbursement procedures and possible conflicts between federal and state interests.

The second general problem area concerns the nature of the audit function itself. One of the characteristics of current procedures is the repeated finding of program deficiencies in subsequent audits of the same entity. Improving the impact of audit reports requires an expanded coverage that includes performance, as well as fiscal and compliance monitoring as part of the audit function. In addition, some notion of accountability needs to be introduced along with enforcement and follow-up procedures for audit recommendations. These two problem areas, audit efficiency and the function of audits, are discussed below along with specific recommendations for improving the role of auditing in the long-term care and disability field.

Audit Efficiency: Duplicate Coverage

The problem of limited audit resources is complicated by the duplication of audit coverage. When numerous groups review the same program, the resulting reports often contain essentially the same findings, with the only differences stemming from variations in scope or perspective. The degree of overlapping in coverage varies but is sufficient to further reduce the amount of total audit resources available. In many cases, several audits may be made of the same operation. Federal, state, and agency program officials, as well as public accountants, may all review one aspect of a program, yet differences in audit approach and content make it extremely difficult for one group to utilize the work of another. The problem is one of allocating the responsibilities and structuring the processes in advance.

As could be expected when two or more entities possess audit responsibilities for the same programs, duplicative auditing of state agencies and programs frequently results. Federal auditors may duplicate the efforts of state program auditors, as well as state central auditors, in the process of auditing for other interests. Federal audits, however, often have a wider scope than states might require for their needs. Federal agencies were first directed to accept as many state audits, or parts of audits, as possible in 1965 by the Office of Management and Budget (OMB) Circular A-73, which was reissued in 1973 as the General Services Administration (GSA) Circular 73-2.[7]

The fact that there has been a lack of overall federal agency compliance with these directives is widely acknowledged by both state and federal agencies. While the cooperation has improved in the past few years, much remains to be done.

An obvious solution which could conserve audit resources as well as minimize interruptions of the day-to-day activities of the audited entity is the concept of a single audit.

The single audit would be an improved audit approach for long-term care and disability audits, one that differentiates the various significant audit concepts and, at the same time, avoids duplication in audit coverage. Fiscal compliance and program auditing are, in fact, simple conceptualizations of different areas of emphasis that actually overlap. It is naive to asssume that one auditor can be assigned to perform compliance audits, another to perform fiscal audits, and still a third to perform program audits without one treading frequently and significantly into the other's land. Equally naive is the notion that financial audits and performance audits should be separated and undertaken by different auditors. Once again, there are so many common features that would require analysis by both auditors that it would be far better to have one comprehensive audit program.

The single audit concept was successfully tested in audits of hospitals by the HEWAA, but it was not continued or adopted elsewhere as a standard unit approach. With federal agencies now more willing than ever to rely on state and local audits to satisfy the requirements of federal assistance programs, and with most states facing serious fiscal crises where both efficiency and effectiveness in state operations are coming under increased scrutiny, there probably has never been a climate more conducive to the development and implementation of a comnprehensive state audit program.

It would be impractical to recommend substantially increasing federal or state audit staffs (even if such an approach is correct in principle). As an alternative, the most feasible source of generating additional audit capacity would seem to be the increased use of certified public accountants. However, some fundamental changes must be made if this is to become a workable reality. To date, most of the audit work involving in-depth compliance and performance reviews has been done by the HEW Audit Agency and the GAO.

Under a "wholesale" concept, most actual field auditing, assuming adequate coverage of all pertinent entities, would be performed by CPAs and by state auditors. The real obstacle to this concept is one of fixing responsibility and accountability where it belongs: namely, where the substantive decisions—medical, administrative, and financial—are made. Under such a policy, the HEW Audit Agency would in effect be a "wholesaler" of audit services rather than operating at the "retail" level performing audits. In this role, the HEWAA would be responsible for identifying areas in the department's long-term care and disability programs that could be audited by public accounting firms and state auditors. These audit groups would utilize specific audit guides prepared and pretested by the Audit Agency. The agency would also monitor the work being performed by public accountants and evaluate its adequacy.

Audit Efficiency: The Reimbursement of Costs

A number of problems arise in attempting to develop a single audit concept and in shifting the burden of its implementation onto the states. While many states have professed a willingness to supplant federal auditors, governors and state central auditors maintain that they cannot afford to extend or take over the responsibility without reimbursement for the costs of performing the audits. An audit acceptable for federal purposes is frequently more extensive than one which is satisfactory to the state. State central audit agencies are unable to hire the manpower, and to command the related support services necessary to do an expanded job, unless they are paid the direct and indirect costs of performing more extensive audits than state law requires.

Federal Management Circular (FMC) 74-4[8] prescribes standards for determining costs applicable to federal grants and contracts with state and local governments. These standards provide a uniform approach for determining allowable grant costs. The circular states that the cost of audits necessary for the administration and management of functions related to grant programs is allowable. State audit costs may be charged against federally assisted programs directly or indirectly. Audit costs may be charged directly when they are related to a specific project or program. Audit costs are generally treated as indirect costs, however, because they usually benefit more than one specific project or program.

According to GAO, most federal agencies allow state audit costs and indirect charges to grant programs. State auditors, however, often have difficulty in having indirect costs approved and accepted by both federal and state program administrators. GAO also found that the auditors of two federal agencies had been successful at contracting with state auditors and making direct payments.[9]

The need for reimbursing state auditors for their help is not the only reason for improving federal reimbursement practices. Even if program administrators were willing to pay for state audit costs, forcing state auditors to rely on them for such payment would jeopardize the auditors' independent standing. Audit independence requires the responsibilities of auditors to be separate from the responsibilities of program administrators. Payment by program administrators to state auditors for audits of federally assisted programs does not adequately separate the responsibilities of these two parties.

"Standards for Audit of Governmental Organizations, Programs, Activities, and Functions," issued by the Comptroller General in 1972, was adopted for federal executive agency audits by FMC 73-2. The standards state that professionals who undertake to audit government activities should be engaged by someone other than the officials responsible for these activities. This practice removes pressures that may exist if the auditor must criticize the performance of those who have engaged him and who are expected to pay him.

Furthermore, there are many people at the federal (and state) level who resist the notion of using a portion of grant money for audits. Program managers, for example, are responsible for approving program-related administrative and audit costs that may be paid out of grant funds. Most program managers candidly admit, however, that they do not want to see the number of dollars in any social program reduced in order to reimburse states for audit costs. Some federal officials have pointed out that there are federal grant programs—such as Revenue Sharing, Disaster Relief, and other programs that provide assistance to states—which the states already audit, although reimbursement is not provided for by law. The federal highway program provides an example of a matching grant program, which, for the most part, is audited at state expense; the enabling legislation did not provide for audit reimbursement.

In several instances, provisions for paying for audit work have been written into program regulations. The money gets diverted from states' central audit offices, however, because the state program managers have control of the funds, and they avoid passing the reimbursable funds through. In some instances the audit funds are allotted to pay the cost of the program manager's own internal auditor staff, or to hire certified public accountants. Through this practice, state program managers avoid turning over to state central auditors or to the state those funds that could be used to strengthen and expand the central audit agencies.

There are several possible ways to circumvent the bureaucratic blockage of funds. One federal agency might extract from grants those funds intended for audit work and give control of the funds to the agency audit office. Another possible approach short of requiring new legislation or a new audit funding grant program, might be to "tag" funds intended to pay audit costs in such a way that they could not be diverted for other program uses.

One reimbursement approach that has been successful for the Environmental Protection Agency (EPA) is the direct contracting approach. EPA's Office of Audit has negotiated contracts with state auditors in California and New York for the audits of construction grants for waste treatment facilities. These audits determine whether the costs incurred agree with grant provisions. The audits are made as single efforts designed to serve both state and federal needs. The potential advantages in using the direct approach are: a) federal auditors may have more assurance that their neds will be satisfied which, in turn, allows them to rely on state audit work as required by FMC 73-2; b) audit coverage is better coordinated; c) direct relations with state auditors are more consistent with the lines of audit responsibility assigned in federal agencies that help to ensure that audit independence is maintained; and d) legal prohibitions against using program funds to pay audit and other indirect costs would not apply if audit costs were reimbursed directly by federal auditors using funds appropriated to them for that purpose.

The primary deterrent to more widespread use of the direct approach is that most federally assisted programs rely on the indirect approach under FMC 74-4 and, therefore, are funded in a manner that does not provide adequate sums for contracting for audits. Funds included in grant programs for paying audit costs under FMC 74-4 would have to be transferred or directly appropriated to the budget of the federal audit group for subsequent direct payment to state auditors or other audit groups. These and other approaches to the reimbursement problem should be explored by audit and legal experts. As long as program managers at either the federal or state level retain discretion over the flow of audit funds, it is unlikely that states will succeed in replacing federal auditors to any great extent.

Audit Efficiency: Federal vs. State Interests

Conflicts between federal and state interests can be a serious problem. Not surprisingly, state governments and the heads of state agencies may interpret federal laws and department long-term care and disability regulations in ways which garner for their state the greatest benefit in dollar terms. In some cases there have been flagrant, and seemingly deliberate, misinterpretations of regulations on the part of state governments and agencies. Such misinterpretations have caused federal agency heads and auditors to fear that federal interests may not be adequately protected if responsibility for auditing is turned over to the states. While this is a legitimate concern, confidence in the "control" afforded by retaining federal auditors is not necessarily the solution. Such confidence would only obscure what may be the real issues: are the federal program managers in headquarters and the field doing their jobs well and are federal program regulations and guidelines written so loosely that they can be easily misinterpreted, deliberately or inadvertently? Furthermore, have adequate internal controls been built into the management and operational processes on which long-term care and disability programs run?

An audit report is actually an ex post facto management tool; it examines what has been done and specifies corrective measures. Looking at the control problem from that perspective raises a question about the efficacy of federal program management. One could argue that the transfer of audits to a state central audit operation from federal agency auditors or their state counterparts might spur better federal management. It could result in: a) more vigilant, effective program management on the part of both federal and state managers; b) fewer cases of deliberate or inadvertent misinterpretation of regulations; c) fewer cases of federal overpayment that result in long, costly battles between federal and state governments. The ultimate impact of the programmatic and organizational developments arising from continuing efforts to redefine the state audit function remains uncertain. Nonetheless, it is clearly evident that state auditing could be an effective tool in obtaining increased audit coverage of long-term care and disability programs.

The Audit Function

Although this chapter is specifically directed at audit deficiencies in long-term care and disability programs, it is also concerned with the broader subject of achieving better program accountability through audit. There is a general consensus that to date, audit findings have not helped to bring about any substantive improvement in overall program performance. To improve the impact of the audit function, a major change in audit policy is required. Three important components of the new policy are the concept of performance auditing, effective audit follow-up procedures, and better coordination between auditing and evaluation.

Performance Auditing

Each fiscal year, federal and state auditors develop "annual work plans." These work plans spell out in some detail the entities and functions to be reviewed during the year. As indicated by the foregoing survey of the audit universe and HEWAA coverage, there is a sizable gap between available audit resources and workload. As a result, audits of the department's long-term care and disability programs are performed on a cyclical basis—every two, three, or four years—on the basis of relative risk. To insure proper accountability, a broad scope audit of each audit "entity" should be conducted every two years, depending on the sensitivity of the audit area, prior audit findings, and the amount of federal funds involved. The audit would cover the fiscal, compliance, and performance of operations regardless of the source of funding.

Performance auditing, or program auditing, is not nearly as well known outside the audit community as fiscal and compliance auditing. The objective of a program audit is to test additional elements of the management control system and to collect other evidence to support an evaluation of the effectiveness of programs in achieving their intended or desired objectives.

There are really two parts or aspects to this type of an audit. First, the auditor must identify and evaluate the various elements of management control to judge their effectiveness in enabling management to measure its own progress toward achieving the program's objectives. Second, the auditor conducts an examination to determine the reliability of the data included in management reports which disclose the program's accomplishment.

Because the concept of performance audit is so new, there are relatively few such audits being done by nonfederal auditors. The HEWAA is very knowledgeable in the conduct of performance audits, and should be able to accommodate any type of evaluation effort. It should be noted that the criteria used in performance audits are established by program personnel, not audit personnel. In addition, there is a large body of evidence available which indicates that self-evaluation by program personnel is not an objective approach.

Audit Follow-Up:

Although the HEWAA and GAO have procedures for follow-up, the primary responsibility for action and follow-up on audit recommendations rests with management. The department currently has in place a follow-up system that includes pre-release procedures wherein audit findings and recommendations are discussed with operating agency officials prior to report issuance. The purpose of these procedures is to foster agreement upon the findings and the corrective actions to be taken. The department's system also calls for annual audit follow-up plans wherein each operating agency identifies significant issues raised as a result of audit, along with actions planned to resolve those issues, including milestone progress reporting dates. The HEWAA is responsible for ensuring that the above procedures are carried out. But the department's poor record in enforcing violations in all of its programs obtains also in the area of audit findings. The position that some federal and state officials take on the question of audit findings is, "so what, in a few months the whole thing will be forgotten." Unfortunately, in too many cases these officials are right.

A good control system will require management officials to evaluate the effectiveness of actions taken on audit recommendations. One procedure they might adopt would be to request, at regular intervals, status reports on efforts to comply with audit recommendations. These reports would be prepared for the information of management officials and auditors alike. Also, provision should be made for regular inquiry into whether proposed corrective actions have been taken and have proved effective. Responsibility for such follow-ups should be with management officials, with participation by the auditors. One of the problems in achieving timely action on audit findings and recommendations is the turnover in senior officials within the department. Top management officials must be reminded on a regular basis that audit-related matters should be handled on a priority basis and not be put aside until there is a dramatic and much publicized breakdown.

To ensure timely and effective follow-up action on audit findings requires an ongoing commitment by top management. The recurrence of deficiencies detected by audits indicates the commitment has not been established. Striving for ways to increase and obtain more in-depth coverage of long-term care and disability programs will prove futile if the results of audits are not properly utilized. The following recommendations are aimed at establishing an effective procedure for following-up on audit findings.

First, the official responsible for implementing audit recommendations should be named in the audit report. The deadline for completing recommended action should also be identified.

Second, an official in the office of the secretary should be designated to monitor and coordinate the actions of agency, regional, and state officials in implementing audit recommendations.

Third, HEWAA should be provided with a staff sufficient in number to determine whether state agencies and other audit entities have implemented the actions necessary to correct reported deficiencies.

Fourth, the reasons for the high incidence of repeat audit findings should be determined. For example, audit recommendations related to repeat findings may be impractical, politically unacceptable, or in conflict with the attitudes of program managers.

Fifth, federal funds should be withheld from states that do not comply with reasonable audit recommendations.

Audit and Evaluation

Auditing, of course, does not function in a vacuum, and it cannot logically be isolated from the administrative, fiscal, evaluative, and related legislative and program requirements and problems that are part of the management of long-term care and disability programs. Also significant are the differences in focus and approach of the various audit entities operating in the public sector. It is quite clear that there are substantial differences of opinion about the role of audit in the evaluation of management practices in long-term care and disability programs. To date, the various audit groups looking at long-term care and disability programs have done very little to coordinate their work with similar work being done through in-house and contract evaluation. On the other hand, little has been done to feed back the results of evaluation to the audit groups. Close formal coordination of audit and evaluation could improve the end-products resulting from audit and evaluation efforts. Coordination could also help to overcome the problem of access-to-records that many contract evaluation efforts have encountered when doing work at state and local levels. Since the HEWAA has access, through legislation, to most state and local records pertaining to federally supported programs, the data needed in many contract evaluations could be obtained through audit.

Finally, this type of coordination could assist evaluation in obtaining hard data—data that have been verified by an independent entity at the "grass roots" level.

There are four general types of evaluation of long-term care and disability programs for which audits could provide valuable input.

Substantive impact evaluations attempt to measure the impact department programs have upon stated objectives. This type of evaluation seeks to determine what the program accomplishes, how these accomplishments compare to program goals, and how much is spent by the program in attempting to realize its goals. The purpose of such evaluation is primarily to provide information for major policy formulation.

Relative effectiveness evaluations compare the effectiveness of two or more major policy strategies or approaches in attaining ultimate objectives within a major program. These studies are designed to help department officials and program managers select the most effective mix of services to maximize a program's total impact—for example, the mix of skilled training, remedial education, and job search assistance in a manpower program.

Efficiency or management evaluations measure the operating efficiency of national programs. These studies are intended primarily to help program managers achieve the most efficient deployment of available resources, rather than to help policy officials arrive at major decisions affecting the scope and focus of the national programs.

Project evaluations entail any of the three preceding types as well as project rating—comparing the effectiveness of one or more individual projects to the outcome of others. Project evaluations are directed toward individual, locally based projects that are components of a national program; they are not necessarily intended to yield conclusions regarding the impact or efficiency of the total national program.

A good example of the type of coordination that can be undertaken between auditing and evaluation is the VR pilot project. The Office of the Assistant Secretary for Planning and Evaluation (ASPE) and the HEW Audit Agency (HEWAA) are currently engaged in a joint audit evaluation of Title I, Section 102 of the Vocational Rehabilitation Act. Section 102 requires the secretary to ensure that the individualized written rehabilitation plan is jointly developed by the VR counselor or coordinator and the handicapped person, and that the plan meets the requirements of Section 102. Thus far, the department has failed to develop regulations concerning Section 102, but the lack of regulations should not have deterred the states from attempting to administer their VR programs according to legislative intent.

To obtain the knowledge and data needed to develop the regulations, the department has elected to use the resources of its Audit Agency in conjunction with an independent contractor. The Audit Agency will be designated "project manager" and the contractor will work under the agency's control and direction during all phases of the project. The objectives of the ASPE-sponsored project are to: determine the responsiveness of VR agency administrators and professionals in complying with the legislative provisions of Section 102; document differences in state interpretation and practices under Section 102; ascertain the reasonableness and validity of key statistical data used by management personnel to evaluate the effectiveness of the VR program; and provide feedback on client expectations and behavior, including more frequent resort to litigation.[10] The results of this pilot project should be evaluated and, if appropriate, the project should be used as a model for future audit/evaluation efforts.

Summary

The recommendations offered in this section are aimed at expanding the role played by the audit function in the performance of long-term care and disability programs. Audit agencies should assume broader responsibility than they have at present and should undertake performance monitoring in addition to fiscal and program compliance. Secondly, resources should be more efficiently utilized by consolidating audit efforts into a single audit mechanism at the state level. The single audit concept, however, requires a method by which funds for the reimbursement of costs flow directly to states' central audit offices. Finally, the findings of audits must be able to be translated into improved program performance. This objective can be achieved by establishing well-defined follow-up procedures that include the use of a penalty approach to reduce the incidence of recurring audit findings and the identification of those to be held accountable for implementing corrections and reforms. In addition, the active role of the audit function can be further enhanced by coordinating audit work with the work undertaken by evaluation teams.

NOTES

1. U.S., Department of Health, Education, and Welfare, *HEW Audit Agency Annual Budget Summary* (March 1975), p. 3.

2. "Audit of Federal Operations and Programs by Executive Branch Agencies," *Federal Management Circular*, FMC 73-2 (September 27, 1973).

3. Most long term care and disability programs contain legislative provisions that authorize and/or require periodic audit of program operations. In addition, the HEWAA has established agreements with certain agencies that call for periodic review of specific programs or functions on a cyclical basis—usually three years. See HEW Audit Agency Annual Workplan, FY 1976, pp. 16–17.

4. U.S., Department of Health, Education, and Welfare, *Summary Report on Audit of Medicaid Administrative Costs in Sixteen States* (HEW Audit Agency, 1969).

5. A summary of GAO's major audit activities is contained in the GAO Report on the *History of Rising Costs of the Medicare and Medicaid Programs and Attempts to Control These Costs: 1966–1975, MOND-76-93* (Washington, D.C.: U.S. General Accounting Office, February 1976).

6. U.S., General Accounting Office, *Review of Controls over the Quality and Costs of Laboratory Services under Four Federally Funded Health Programs* (1977).

7. Federal Management Circular 73-2, *Audit of Federal Operations and Programs by Executive Branch Agencies*, p. 4. "Reports prepared by nonfederal auditors will be used in lieu of federal audits if the reports and supporting work papers are available for review by the federal agencies, if testing by federal agencies indicates the audits in accordance with generally accepted auditing standards, and if the audits otherwise meet the requirements of the federal agencies."

8. Comptroller General of the United States, *Problems in Reimbursing State Auditors for Audits of Federally Assisted Programs* (June 25, 1975).

9. Ibid.

10. U.S., Department of Health, Education, and Welfare. Audit Agency. *Consolidated Report on the Administration of the Vocational Rehabilitation Program*, ACN 15-70300 (1977).

6

PATIENT-RELATED REIMBURSEMENT
FOR LONG-TERM CARE

Thomas J. Walsh

In setting reimbursement rates which are adequate but not excessive, the states must next come to terms with the question, "How should payments be differentiated to reflect varying levels of need?" While most would agree that the overall level of reimbursement must be appropriate to prevent either excessive or insufficient entry, it should be recognized that inadequate differentiation among patients will lead to the same undesirable consequences for subgroups of patients. For example, a flat rate for all ICF patients would probably create a rush for patients who require little care, while making it difficult for patients who need more extensive services to obtain adequate care.

Thus in establishing reimbursement policy for long-term care, four major questions arise concerning whether reimbursement should vary with patient condition:

1. Do significant variations in patient condition and patient need exist within any categories of long-term care?

2. If such differences do exist, do they imply important differences in the cost of caring for patients?

3. Can differential payments for patients with unequal needs be incorporated into a cost-related reimbursement system?

4. Is the inclusion of reimbursement differentials to compensate for differential cost desirable or undesirable on the whole?

In general, reimbursement for differential needs would be accomplished by applying a valid patient assessment tool to patients at intake, relating cost of care to the patient assessment, and stratifying reimbursement for patients with different levels of need according to the results of the assessment tool.

The present paper will discuss attempts to relate patient assessment to reimbursement in Illinois and describe two methodologies employed in that effort. We will begin with a brief history of patient-related reimbursement in the state, focusing on the Illinois "point count system," and then discuss the adaptation of this system to cost-related reimbursement. We will also describe an alternative methodology employed where the point count was inapplicable. Finally, we will summarize experience in Illinois and point up implications for further development of reimbursement systems.

HISTORY OF PATIENT ASSESSMENT IN ILLINOIS

Illinois is one of the few states in the nation that has used patient assessment as an integral part of its reimbursement systems. For the past ten years, the state has used a system commonly referred to as the "point system" to purchase long-term care. That system has three components—a base rate, a point count reimbursement, and "add-on" payments for special services. The base component is a flat rate paid for all patients regardless of their needs, and is expected to compensate for provision of basic services required by all patients. This is augmented by a payment designed to compensate for care rendered to patients with needs above the minimum level. Differential need is measured by a patient evaluation system commonly referred to as the point system. (A summary of the Illinois Point Count System is available from the author on request.)

Under the point count system patients are awarded "points" or scores for each condition that requires services not usually provided to all patients. For example, a patient who needs assistance in eating is given three points, while a patient who must be tube fed receives eight, and those who require no assistance receive none. Patients are evaluated by caseworkers of the Illinois Department of Public Aid. Each point adds $6.00 or $5.00 per month to the reimbursement, depending on whether or not the facility is in Chicago.

Finally, facilities which have programs certified by the Illinois Department of Public Health receive a flat reimbursement for each patient day for special activity programs, rehabilitation nursing, and social rehabilitation.

The essential part of the reimbursement system for our purposes is its relation to patient condition and needs as represented by the point count system. It represents a type of patient-related reimbursement similar to what might be envisioned as an application of the Patient Appraisal and Care Evaluation (PACE) developed by the Office of Long-Term Care in the U.S. Department of Health, Education, and Welfare. The pertinent question, then, is whether or not experience with the point count has interesting implications for patient-related reimbursement in general, and whether or not that experience has been generally favorable or unfavorable.

The Illinois experience with patient-related reimbursement has indicated several major problems. These include severe difficulties in administering the reimbursement system, problems with completeness of the assessment tool, and difficulty in accurately relating services to reimbursement.

Probably the most unappealing aspect of tying reimbursement to patient assessment is the administrative complexity that necessarily accompanies such a policy. First, the patient assessment tool must be applied to each patient not once, but as frequently as substantial changes in service needs might occur. In Illinois, SNF patients are reevaluated every 60 days, while ICF patients are reevaluated quarterly. Even for a patient assessment tool as simple as the point assessment, the expense of administration approaches $4 million each year. This cost can be minimized, of course, by maintaining as simple an assessment tool as possible.

A second difficulty with the administration of such a reimbursement system has emerged. Because patients must be periodically reevaluated, a very large number of caseworkers must be employed in the evaluation, and all of the inconsistencies commonly encountered in autonomous evaluations by a large number of individuals can be expected. In the best case, differences of interpretation of regulations will result in differential payments. Also, animosity or friendship between caseworkers and operators will result in arbitrary differences in reimbursement.

In the worst case, the power given the caseworker places that person in an ideal position to receive bribes—and the amount of money involved is substantial. A change of only one point for each patient can bring the owner of a 100-bed facility $6,000 to $7,000 per year, and cost the system as a whole as much as $3 million annually.

In short, the autonomy and authority conferred on caseworkers by patient-related reimbursement introduces in the reimbursement system all of the human elements of inconsistency, arbitrariness, and corruption. Therefore, the simpler and more objective the assessment tool, the smaller the problem posed by this set of elements. In fact, a recent evaluation of regional differences in point scores indicated a variance of approximately 15 percent among regions in the state. Because the regions are large, it is unlikely that variance in patient condition can account for this variation, and the variations probably reflect differences in regional policies or caseworker proclivities in various regions.

In addition to citing administrative problems, many claim that a simple patient assessment tool such as the point count system cannot capture all of the needs that can be expected to affect costs of operation. In this case, those patients whose needs are not well represented will have difficulty finding placement. The solution to this objection is obviously to expand the assessment tool. However, the more complex the tool the greater the administrative expense and the greater the reliance on the caseworkers' capacity to evaluate patient needs fairly.

Perhaps the most important objection to patient-related reimbursement in Illinois, however, has been that in the past point count reimbursement has not been empirically related to the cost of providing care. At present, the relationship of reimbursement to cost of care is only approximate, and it may have created a series of incentives contrary to the best interests of the patients. For example, suppose that the actual cost of feeding a patient in bed is $2.00 each day, and points worth $2.50 each day are awarded for feeding a patient in bed. The operator has an incentive to keep as many patients as possible bedridden. Thus, the charge has been leveled that the point system discourages the successful treatment or restoration of patients.

Secondly, given the federal mandate for cost-related reimbursement, the patient assessment tool must in the future be related to the costs of providing care, and this may be an expensive and difficult procedure. If one must conduct an engineering-time/motion study, the time required to develop a cost-related system can be substantial. Furthermore, difficulties in estimating the impact of joint product situations (for example, turning and treating bed sores at the same time), and normal differences in time required for a given activity across facilities will often result in a substantial variance in the estimate.

Once we have noted these disadvantages, we can argue that the application of a patient assessment tool to the reimbursement system has one overwhelming advantage—it allows us to tailor reimbursement to patients at one end of the continuum who are mobile, lucid, and able to care for most of their daily living needs autonomously, as well as to those at the other end who are completely immobile, senile, and/or have significant medical problems. Although a high priority in Illinois was to supplant the point count system when developing a cost-related system as mandated by federal statute, and though this goal was announced by the governor himself, we found it impossible to eliminate that system without having some alternative assessment tool in place. (The range of patient needs, and the cost differences associated with differential need, were too great to be included in one flat rate system, or even two or three flat rate categories.) Point scores actually awarded to patients ranged from less than 5 to 25 for patients in ICF levels of care, and from 20 to over 50 for patients in skilled care. The answer to the first question posed above appears to be that substantial differences in the need for care do exist among patients in the same level of care.

THE REIMBURSEMENT APPROACH

Having determined that differences in patients' needs exist, we must next inquire whether those differences have major cost implications. How will patient assessments, which are generally a detailed listing of services required by the patient, be related to the cost of operating a long-term care facility? There are two competing methodologies that may be employed: (1) the estimation of cost relationships by standard statistical methods; and (2) the estimation of service-time-cost relationships through the use of cost data applied to time-motion studies. This latter approach will be referred to as an "engineering" approach and the former as a statistical approach. Both approaches were applied in Illinois in developing its long-term care reimbursement system.

The Statistical Approach

The statistical approach requires development of a theoretical framework as the first step in estimating cost relationships. The theoretical model will then be translated into a series of quantifiable variables and related to observed costs.

In formulating theoretical relationships, we begin with the most traditional case, that of the proprietary long-term care operator seeking maximization of profit. We assume that such a producer competes in a monopolistically competitive market for private patients, in which price is a function of quantity offered and the extent to which the producer can differentiate his product by providing "amenities"—quality of service above the required for operation. These amenities may be related to medical care, such as minimal waiting time when nursing services are required, or may be represented by the quality of living standards. Thus,

$$P = P(Q,A)$$

where: P = the private market price
α = the proportion of services offered to private patients
Q = the quantity of services produced
A = the amenity level

Both the quantity of services and the amenity level are assumed to be related to levels of input which we, for convenience, will assume to be capital, K, and labor, L. Inputs used to improve the quality above the minimum required level of care will be labeled K_a and L_a, while those used to increase quantity will be labeled K and L. Thus,

$$Q = Q(K, L)$$

$$A = A(K_a, L_a)$$

While the producer is assumed to be a monopolistic competitor in the market for private patients, he faces a fixed reimbursement for Medicaid patients. In this case, price variation is not a factor in attracting patients, but the amenity level may be. It is assumed that the producer is prevented from discriminating against Medicaid patients in providing amenities. This would be consistent with the assumption that all patients in the same section of the long-term care facility receive equivalent services.

The objective function of the long-term care provider, as described above, is assumed to be the revenue function:

$$P(\alpha Q(K,L), A(K_a,L_a)) \, \alpha Q(K,L) + M(1 - \alpha)Q(K,L)$$

where: M = the Medicaid reimbursement rate
$(1 - \alpha)$ = the proportion of Medicaid patients

In seeking to maximize profits, the producer is constrained by the cost function:

$$C = WL + WL_a + IK + IK_a$$

where: W = the wage rate
I = the implicit rental rate on capital

The standard technique to determine the profit maximizing conditions under constraints is the introduction of the Lagrange multiplier. The Lagrangian described by this system has six unknowns or decision variables: the labor input to quantity, the labor input to quality, the capital input to quantity, the capital input to quality, the proportion of output to be devoted to private versus Medicaid patients, and the Lagrangian multiplier, λ. Differentiating with respect to these six variables provides six first-order conditions that must be met for profits to be maximized.

$$\partial \pi / \partial L = P'_q Q'_L \alpha Q + P \alpha Q'_L + M(1 - \alpha)Q'_L = \lambda W \tag{1}$$

$$\partial \pi / \partial L_a = P'_A A'_{L_a} \partial Q = \lambda W \tag{2}$$

$$\partial \pi / \partial K = P'_a / Q'_K \alpha Q + P \alpha Q'_K + M(1 - \alpha)Q'_K = \lambda I \tag{3}$$

$$\partial \pi / \partial K_a = P'_A A'_{K_a} \alpha Q = \lambda I \tag{4}$$

$$\partial \pi / \partial \alpha = P'_\alpha \alpha Q + P = M \quad \text{where: } P'_\alpha < 0 \tag{5}$$

$$\partial \pi / \partial \lambda = C = W(L + L_a) + I(K + K_a) \tag{6}$$

Verbally, the six conditions specify that the marginal unit of labor (capital) used to increase quantity must result in marginal revenue from private and public patients equal to the wage (interest rate) times λ. Similarly, the marginal cost of increasing amenities must equal the value of marginal revenue from private patients brought about by the change in amenity level. Third, the marginal return from a unit of labor (capital) used in increasing quantity must equal the marginal return from a unit of labor (capital) used to increase amenities. Finally, the public-private patient mix must be chosen so that the marginal revenue from private patients equals the Medicaid rate.

In terms of the cost function the above analysis implies, cost will be a function of the quantity of services provided, the amenity level, and input prices W and I. That is,

$$C = C(Q, A, W, I)$$

or

$$C/Q = C(Q, A, W, I).$$

The analysis is complicated if it is extended to the case of nonprofit or county nursing facilities. Included in the objective functions of those facilities may be an intrinsic preference for serving Medicaid patients, for a level of amenities well above minimum standards, and for service to constituent populations. In this case the maximization problem changes slightly, but the analogous theoretical construct would be maximizing the subjective value of possible output subject to the constraint that revenues are not less than costs. It can be demonstrated that under these assumptions the decision variables remain the same, and the determinants of the cost function remain unchanged. What one expects is a set of equilibrium values that differ between the voluntary, county, and proprietary sectors, because the objective functions of each of the sectors are in some way unique to that sector.

In estimating the cost function generally described above, it was assumed that the elasticities of substitution between labor and capital are close to zero, and that the effects of differences in input prices can be treated by deflating cost figures to a common level by means of a price index. Such an index was constructed using wage and salary data submitted by facilities on their cost reporting forms. After discussion with industry representatives and in the absence of reliable interregional indexes, we assumed that wholesale prices of nonlabor inputs were approximately constant across the state.

The amenity level provided was somewhat difficult to represent, since a simple representation as input levels for each patient would have resulted in a trivial estimation. On the other hand, amenity level in terms of outputs is virtually impossible to measure comprehensively. Therefore, we chose four variables to represent amenities: an indicator of the general level of nursing quality provided in the facility; the proportion of Public Aid patients served by the facility; a binary variable representing county ownership; and a binary variable representing voluntary ownership. The coefficient of the variable representing proportion of Public Aid patients is expected to represent the cost of average amenity levels required to attract Medicaid patients. The interpretation of the binary variables as being related to amenity levels is somewhat arbitrary, being based on the assumption that operators of such facilities will have a preference for amenities. An alternative interpretation is that variance in costs related to ownership differences will reflect management efficiency.

The variable representing quality of care provided was a scaled variable constructed from reviews of licensing inspections, medical reviews, and private complaints against the facilities. These reviews include assessment of food, quality of medical care, quality of housekeeping, and compliance with housing standards. The maximum score possible for this variable, 50 points, indicated that no violations, deficiencies, or reasonably substantiated complaints were in evidence.

The validity of this quality variable was tested by drawing a sample of facilities and scoring each facility. Caseworkers and Department of Public Health field personnel were then asked to evaluate the sample facilities in their region as good, fair to good, and poor. All facilities scoring above 45 points were uniformly classed as "good" by the caseworkers and field representatives. Virtually all ratings of those scored below 35 were poor. While the cardinal accuracy of the scores may be questioned, we believe the scoring represents a reasonably reliable ordinal measure. Furthermore, it allowed us to consider a dimension for which virtually no objective measures exist.

Two variables were used to describe the nature of the care being provided in each facility—a dimension of product differentiation. The average point count in each facility was used to represent the level of need of patients receiving care. In addition. the percentage of patients being provided skilled care was used as a complementary index of the severity of patient needs.

Finally, three variables were used to represent elements of management efficiency in each facility. Licensed capacity was used to represent possible economies or diseconomies of scale in long-term care facilities. Secondly, a variable expressing capacity utilization represented the extent to which facilities were underutilized. Finally, whether or not one or more of the owners actually worked in the facility was included in the expectation that administrators with a financial stake in the operation of the facility would tend to reduce operation expenses.

Intuitively, this model may be thought of as a cost function for a series of products, produced in the same facility but fairly independent of each other. The basic output would be one day of ICF care that meets minimum standards. To this basic product the administrator may add a set amount to produce a day of skilled care that meets minimum standards, an amount to produce increments in care or noncare amenities that are in excess of required minimums, and a set amount for each service indicated by points assigned to patients. Finally, efficiency factors are assumed to be related to the volume of product being delivered.

The equation used to estimate the cost is:

$$TC = a_0 + a_1Q + a_2SK + a_3PT + a_4PT^2 + \sum_{i=5}^{8} a_iA_iQ + \sum_{j=1}^{3} a_jE_jQ$$

or

$$CPD = a'_0 + a'_1 + a'_2SK/Q + a'_3PT/Q + a'_4PT^2/Q + \sum_{i=5}^{8} a'_iA_i + \sum_{i=5}^{3} a'_jE_j$$

where:
  TC = Total operating cost
  CPD = Operating cost each patient day
  Q = Number of patient days
  SK = Number of skilled days
  PT = Total point count
  A_i = Amenity level
  E_j = Efficiency factor j

In estimating the cost function we regressed operating cost for each long-term care day on the variables described above. The results are presented in Table 6.1. As the table indicates, both the signs and magnitudes of the coefficients are consistent with intuitive expectations. The most interesting result from the point of view of one interested in relating patient assessment to reimbursement is that both the point count assessment score and the variable indicating skilled care are important and statistically significant predictors of operating cost. In addition both county and voluntary facilities are substantially more expensive than proprietary institutions, while the proportion of Medicaid patients is inversely related to costs. Finally, our quality indicator is positively correlated with costs, and can be said to differ from zero at the .95 level of confidence. What emerges is that patients' condition as measured by point scores and the level of care in which patients are placed both have important implications for the cost of providing care. A skilled patient is estimated to increase costs by \$2.73 each day, while each additional point awarded a patient is expected to increase costs by an amount that varies according to the point score. The differential cost of caring for a patient with five points as opposed to that of caring for a patient with 25 points would be estimated as \$5.20 per day—

TABLE 6.1

Regression Results for the Cost Equation

Variable	Coefficient	Standard Error	t
Average Point Score	.5065	.1294	3.91
Average Point Score Squared	−.0082	.0030	2.73
Percent Skilled Patients	3.0200	.8963	3.37
Quality Score	.1123	.0632	1.78
Percent Medicaid Patients	−.8348	1.101	.833
County Ownership Binary	5.1671	.7075	7.30
Non-Profit Binary	2.6799	.7419	3.61
Capacity in Number of Beds	−.00002	.00001	1.93
Percent of Capacity Utilization	−9.5674	2.6367	3.62
Working Owner Binary	−1.2971	.6460	2.07
Constant	16.38		
R^2	.5689		
Standard Error of the Estimate	2.746		
F Statistic	21.5884		
N	136		

Source: Compiled by the authors.

approximately 33 percent of the average operating cost of Illinois ICF facilities. This represents a substantial cost and a substantial incentive to accept low-need patients over high-need patients in a flat-rate system.

Having determined that important differences between patients do exist, and that they have important cost implications, we can proceed to estimate the reimbursement level required to compensate for patient differences. The empirical estimate of cost relationships is used to determine the cost implications of each variable in the equation, and then only those variables that are desirable from a policy viewpoint are included in the actual reimbursement equation.

For example, the results indicate that voluntary and county facilities are more expensive than proprietary facilities. Since there is no compelling reason to believe that the state shares the objective function of either of these groups, nor to assume that the state should share in any inefficiencies that the higher costs represent, these coefficients may be ignored. Similarly, the state has no preference for providing a level of amenities unrelated to patient care that is in excess of that required to attract Medicaid patients.

Accordingly, the proportion of Medicaid patients is assumed to be 1.0. However, the state does have a preference for high quality care. In Illinois, a hypothetical score of 45 points was assigned to each facility, and the effect of that score level on expense was added to the reimbursement system. In effect, this represents a policy of reimbursing each facility an adequate amount to allow it to reach what regulatory personnel regard as a good level of care.

In terms of management efficiency, the results suggest that size has a precisely measured but trivial effect on costs, and can be disregarded. Utilization of capacity has an important and precisely measured effect on costs. However, reimbursement for operation at less than 90 percent of capacity would probably encourage wasteful employment of resources except in the case where demand is growing rapidly. Thus, in Illinois, all facilities are to be reimbursed as though they operate at a target level of occupancy equal to 93 percent, the current average capacity utilization. Finally, if we assume that the working owner represents the ideal in efficiency, we might include that coefficient in determining reimbursement.

All of the factors discussed thus far will be estimated as constant across facilities. For example, county ownership equals 0, occupancy equals .93, quality equals 45, and so forth. Accordingly, all such factors can be combined with the constant. What remains are those variables representing level of patient need—the point count scores, and the skilled care indicator. In general, the reimbursement system that follows is:

$$\text{Reimbursement} = K + \alpha_1 \text{ points} + \alpha \text{ skilled care}$$

$$= 10.08 + .54 \text{ points} - .008 \text{ points}^2 + 3.02 \text{ skilled care binary}$$

Thus, when a patient enters long-term care, he would be assessed to determine his score in assessment points and whether or not he requires skilled care. Once these determinations have been made, the caseworker bills according to the above formula. Practically, of course, the formula must be deflated for regional differences through application of the above mentioned price index and translated into a table for easy reference by caseworkers.

The Engineering Approach

While the statistical approach offers a good deal of flexibility in formulating reimbursement policy, it may not always be the preferred approach.

It may be desirable to obtain more detailed information on the relation betwen specific patient conditions and cost of care. Or the historical data required to estimate statistical relationships may be unavailable. In these cases a more structured engineering approach may be preferable.

One such model was employed in Illinois in an attempt to determine reimbursement for program services in facilities serving developmentally disabled children. Providers of care and state program monitors agreed that the point count, while possibly suited to a medically needy geriatric population, was not appropriate as a means of evaluating the developmentally disabled. Consequently, a task force developed an alternative patient assessment tool for this population.*

The first step in formulation of the assessment tool was identification of needs likely to be encountered with the developmentally disabled population. The needs include activities of daily living (ADL) skills such as eating and mobility, medical services such as medications and injections, and program services such as physical therapy, neurological development and sensory stimulation as well as communication/speech, hearing, and language development.

The second step in the process was identification of the probable frequency values for each need, the number and type of personnel involved in meeting the need, and the time input required from each of the personnel. To this end, time-motion studies were conducted in three facilities, and the results were used to calculate the following relationship:

$$\text{Staff Time i} = \text{Number of staff} \times (\text{frequency/month}) \times (\text{duration}) \times \text{group factor}$$

where:

Staff Time i = time required to serve a patient with need i over a one-month period

Frequency = the expected number of times services will be needed in a month

Duration = the number of hours one service is expected to be required

Group Factor = the reciprocal of the average number of clients served at the same time (For example, activities may be conducted with a group of four, so that only ¼ of the staff time is assigned to one recipient.)

While this formula provides an estimate of the time involved, it does not address itself to the cost of the service. This is accomplished through the application of a set of multipliers based on wage indexes. Wage data were

---

*The tool is available from the author.

used to construct an index of average wage by type of staff, with aides serving as the base. For example, if on average, aides receive $2.50 an hour, RNs $5.00, and therapists $4.00, the index would express aides as 1.0, RNs as 2.0, and therapists as 1.6. The staff time estimate presented above is then multiplied by the index representing the type of labor involved in performance of each task to convert the time estimate to a relative cost estimate which should be constant over time:

$$\text{Service Cost Index} = \Sigma(\text{staff index} = i \times \text{number of staff}) \times \text{frequency} \times \text{duration} \times \text{group factor} \times \text{nonlabor factor}$$

Finally, a factor representing nonlabor costs of providing the service is included. For example, if labor is estimated to be 80 percent of the direct cost of the service, the nonlabor multiplier would be 1.25.

The approach has the advantage that, if the measurements are accurate, the reimbursement mechanism needs little adjustment over time. To obtain the cost of any services, the Service Cost Index is multiplied by the base wage rate—the average wage of the aides. As long as relative wages remain approximately constant and no changes in care technology occur, the index can be updated by simple application of the average aide's wage.

While the engineering approach has some appeal, however, the estimates it provided in practice were not consistent with observed program costs. First, the level of expenditure indicated by the engineering approach averaged approximately 15 percent above that reported by facilities. Secondly, the pattern of expenditures across facilities indicated by the index was not consistent with reported expenses or with the expectations of state program monitors. That is, personnel with responsibility for monitoring care being provided by these institutions concluded that in some cases facilities with simple programs were assigned higher reimbursement than facilities with much more complex programs serving more difficult clients. The implication is that the staff time factors were misestimated in the time-motion studies.

Whether these problems represent a misapplication of the time-motion technique or an intrinsic fault of such an approach is difficult to assess. The engineering approach is usually based on a relatively small sample, and differences between facilities in the time required to perform a given task may be substantial. Furthermore, some possible economies of performing tasks in groups rather than individually may not be immediately apparent when measurement is directed at isolated tasks. The result will be overestimation of expense. At any rate, it seems imperative that the results of such estimates be tested against observed cost levels as well as by comparison with the judgement of those familiar with the operation of the facilities being examined.

SUMMARY AND CONCLUSION

These results indicated that from an economic point of view, differentiation of reimbursement according to patient need is both justified and feasible. The statistically based cost estimates appear to be reasonably precise, and they predict reimbursement levels that are compatible with both the level and distribution of costs observed in cost reports. In addition, application of this system in Illinois has indicated that acceptance of the technique by the long-term care industry is fairly good. The procedures tend to look like a black box to the industry, but to this point there has been no substantial disagreement with the distribution of reimbursement produced by using the regression coefficients. Problems with the engineering approach are more substantial, but we are proceeding with a reassessment of the staff time/service coefficients in the expectation that better estimates can be obtained.

However, the question remains—is patient-related reimbursement diesirable—and substantial problems still do exist with the application of patient assessment to reimbursement. First, there are problems of proportionality in the point count assessment tool as it now exists. For example, it is not clear that the cost of occasionally providing oxygen is greater than provision of a special diet ordered by a physician, though more points are assigned. In the coming year we will be revising this assessment tool.

Secondly, we are convinced that inconsistencies exist in the application of the tool. Consequently, we are seeking to simplify the tool as much as possible, to express the condition that warrants assignment of points in as objective terms as possible, and finally, to implement a monitoring system that will summarize points assigned by caseworkers, by offices, and by regions. Deviations from normal patterns can be identified and either explained or altered. Inconsistent or subjective application of the point count tool tends to increase the error in measurement of patient condition, and though we believe the error is randomly distributed, the consequence is probably excessive variance in the estimated coefficient. Accordingly, we expect to obtain a more precise estimate of this coefficient in the future.

Finally, while we have included a measure of care quality in our equation to assure that the costs of adequate care are covered, we recognize that there is no incentive in the current system ro assure that such care will actually be provided. Accordingly, reimbursement will not be fully appropriate until it can be adjusted to reward quality. All of the shortcomings in the patient-related reimbursement system developed for Illinois that we have cited here also serve to underscore the difficulty of implementing and administering such a system. This difficulty should be considered in weighing the pros and cons of tying patient assessment to reimbursement. Despite all of these problems, however, failure to reimburse according to patient need will create what appear to be powerful preferences on the part of providers for patients with relatively low needs. As a result, states will either have to reimburse at a level appropriate for the highest level patient or risk shortages of capacity for those patients in the long run. On balance, these long run tradeoffs appear to justify the time and effort required to implement patient-related reimbursement.

7
DESIRED CHANGES IN CURRENT REGULATORY MECHANISMS FROM THE POINT OF VIEW OF A NURSING HOME ADMINISTRATOR

Harvey Wertlieb

The long-term care administrator brings a very different point of view to the discussion of industry regulation. Taking my experience as a guide, I will offer some observations on this subject and make some suggestions for possible changes in regulatory procedures. Before I present my recommendations, however, I would like to consider certain social, historical, and economic developments that have both influenced the position in which long-term care administrators find themselves and shaped their attitudes toward regulation.

GROWTH AND UTILIZATION OF LONG-TERM CARE

I believe it is safe to say that the modern era in long-term care originated with the passing of the Social Security Act of 1935. The act represented the beginning of a social welfare policy, and it set into motion the rapid, sometimes haphazard development of the long-term care industry. This irregular and unplanned approach to meeting the needs of the elderly accelerated in the late 50s and early 60s until the creation of Medicare and Medicaid. The passage of legislation establishing these programs signaled a significant change in emphasis and direction in the long-term care program in the United States.

During the 30 years between 1935 and 1965, monthly social security checks enabled elderly people to pay for services in boarding and rest homes. Demand for these services increased tremendously as the number of elderly increased. Because of advances in modern medicine, increased health care services grew along with social programs. However, while demand and services increased, funds were frequently unavailable to pay for new or better-equipped facilities. Because of insufficient funds and professional disinterest, the quality of services also did not improve in many cases.

At the same time, state and local regulations governing boarding homes and rest homes did not exist or were weak and ineffective. In a sense, the industry developed in a vacuum, removed from public awareness, interest, and perception of need. Like state mental institutions, long-term care facilities were out of sight and therefore out of mind. Licensing and certification programs were implemented on an "as needed" basis. As the public sector recognized a problem, agencies enacted a law or established a licensing category. In addition, very few funds were allocated to implement or enforce these laws.

A quirk in the Social Security Act caused most institutions providing long-term care to develop as proprietary facilities. This has remained true up to the present. Today 76 percent of long-term beds in the United States—or some 852,800 beds—are operated for profit.

This orientation meant that most institutions were operated in a businesslike manner. As the field became more complex and demanding, the small mom and pop nursing homes gave way to the larger, more diversified facilities with experienced management. The tendency of management was to deliver services according to the consumer's ability to pay. Because the majority of persons in these facilities were dependent on Social Security and limited savings, management was not inclined to build better and more expensive facilities or to expand and upgrade their services.

As conditions in the forties deteriorated, and more and more unpleasant situations started coming to the attention of the public officials, intermittent attempts were made to channel new funds into facility development. State and local authorities also began writing regulations to correct specific problems. Still, very little effort was made to fund the implementation of these regulations or to train enforcement agents to carry out their duties.

Federal involvement began to surface in the fifties with the advent of the Hill-Burton and Federal Housing Administration programs, and finally with the Kerr-Mills Old Age Assistance program (the forerunner of Medicare). Although these programs represented positive developments, most of them failed to provide adequate funding for facilities and services. In the long run, they did not make a dent in alleviating the pending problems of a troubled industry. For example, as late as 1964, the State of Maryland was paying only $4.35 per day for patient care.

With the advent of Medicaid and Medicare, federal involvement with the area of long-term care has expanded rapidly. The industry has been unable to match this commitment; funds for improved facilities and services remain scarce. Even today, patient per day payments are less than

TABLE 7.1

Spending for Long-Term Patient Care

Years	(Millions)	Percent of Total National Health Expenditures
1940	$ 28	.7
1950	178	1.5
1965	480	1.9
1965	1,271	3.3
1970	3,818	5.5
1976	10,600	7.6
1980	19,571*	8.3

*Forecast.

Source: Research & Statistics Note #27, Social Security Administration, December 22, 1976.

$20.00 in many states. As the industry has fallen behind in its ability to provide services, the public has become increasingly aware of its needs in the long-term care area and increasingly outspoken in its criticism of the industry. When the failure of some facilities to comply with life safety code regulations came to the attention of the public, it caused considerable outrage; there was little effort on the part of the industry critics to understand the position of the providers who in 1976 lacked the resources to improve outdated facilities. (It should also be noted that most of these alleged deficiencies were paper deficiencies that might be resolved by a different interpretation of the code.) I would like to see some recognition of the fact that the industry has never had adequate funding to meet the demands of society or to respond fully to its criticisms.

The effect of Medicare and Medicaid on the long-term care industry merits more detailed consideration. When Titles 18 and 19 of the Social Security Act were passed by Congress in 1965, it was thought that most of the problems of the industry would be solved by the infusion of millions of dollars of funds into the system.

Table 7.1 shows the results of this massive infusion of monies. The programs were also intended to establish a national standard by which quality care could be measured and to create controls that would ensure the delivery of such care.

There is little doubt that the passage of Titles 18 and 19 had a marked effect, altering the whole course of long-term care in our country in midstream. But this effect was not the anticipated one. The programs created confusion among the public and the industry. They totally disrupted the government structure, which was intended to implement, manage, and enforce the acts. Still, Medicare and Medicaid also had positive effects, which are obvious to many of us:

1. They changed the focus of the previous welfare programs from social care to that of medical care.
2. They shifted the responsibility of providing medical care from the individual or the family to society as a whole. In essence, they made health care a *right*.
3. They established a national set of federal standards enforced by the states; long-term care facilities had the option to participate or not participate.
4. They established a reimbursement system, which in the most complimentary terms I call a *cost less* system.
5. They focused the attentions of the public sector on the inadequacies of the field.

At the height of the Medicare program in 1966–68 only 25 percent of all patients in long-term care facilities received Medicare Part A benefits. Today less than 5 percent of all patients in long-term care facilities receive inpatient benefits. On the other hand, the Medicaid program has gained in importance in the past ten years, so that approximately 65 percent of inpatients are presently covered by this program. Virtually every licensed facility in the country is regulated by standards established by authority of the Titles 18 and 19 laws of 1965, 1972, and 1974. In 1967–68, most long-term care institutions were not able to meet Medicare standards and opted to remain under state licensing, which was less costly and posed fewer compliance problems.

Isolated events, together with the birth of the consumer movement, prodded Congress to enact legislation (Public Law 92-603, 1972) to federalize some aspects of the Medicaid program that had been a state-federal grant-in-aid program. For the first time *all* long-term care facilities that received any federal funds were required to comply with national standards. Failure to comply would lead to the termination of funds. To date, many of the provisions of Public Law 92-603 have yet to be implemented by HEW, including a provision that health care institutions must be paid on a cost-related basis by July 1, 1974.

The 1972 and 1974 laws failed to clarify some of the more confusing provisions of the original legislation. As a consequence, the industry has been unable to deliver the quality of service demanded by the public. Health planning is not working. Professional Standards Review Organizations—organizations concerned with cost containment and quality of care in hospitals—have neglected long-term care and are floundering.

Alternative services are not being developed in an effective way, an acceptable reimbursement system is far from being realized, and we still have not identified the patient we are trying to serve.

Other federal programs, such as the Occupational Safety and Health Administration, civil rights, hiring the handicapped, the energy program, minimum wage and the Administrative Procedures Act, have imposed various kinds of restrictions on the management and operation of long-term care facilities. Despite this, the industry has moved on: improving our facilities, improving our documentation procedures, and improving staff training and professional development. We have also improved our ability to analyze the significance of past and future legislative programs from the point of view of the provider.

We have not, of course, moved fast enough or far enough in the past 12 years to satisfy anyone. The important point is that we have moved forward against great odds, and we hope that we will be allowed to move forward in the future.

SOCIOECONOMIC FACTORS

Today, our society is youth-oriented, but there is evidence that the trend will reverse itself as the aged population expands. There are already more than 20 million people in the country over 65 years of age. By the year 2000, there will be 31.8 million aged or 12.2 percent of the population, and these people will require more and more health and social services.

In light of the growing number of old persons, the long-term care facility can be expected to take on new and more complex roles. At this time it affects only 5 percent of the population over 65, but there is no question that it will affect a larger proportion of persons in the future. Long-term care facilities are also beginning to be utilized in a greater proportion by persons under 65. Long-term care facilities can be hospitals, chronic hospitals, or skilled nursing facilities; they can be residential or hospice, health oriented or socially oriented. Long-term care facilities can be a combination of all or one of these services. They could provide alternative services such as outpatient therapy, home care, day care, meals on wheels, or activities programs. They could provide these services with adequate quality, with flexibility, and in a cost-effective manner. Better linkages could be and should be established between all sectors of the health delivery system including the public and private sectors.

There are three major reasons why the long-term care sector has been unable to provide these alternative services. The public lacks any substantial knowledge of long-term care, at the same time that its general attitude toward the system of care is negative. Every effort is being made by opinion leaders and consumer advocates to bring down the institutions as a viable living environment and treatment center and to encourage the creation of duplicate services in other settings. The intention of the advocates is to keep people in their homes regardless of the cost.

The professions have failed to become involved in understanding and treating the problems of the aged. Our medical, nursing, and other disciplines have totally neglected the geriatric field. It is only in the past few years that we see the medical education institutions even beginning to respond to the need for a geriatric curriculum. While the response is in its earliest phase, however, almost all new regulations pertaining to long-term care institutions require trained, experienced, licensed, or certified personnel to staff the facilities. Given the limited number of persons who have the training or experience to fill these jobs, the regulations are unrealistic. There is still too little support from the professionals to direct and operate long-term care programs effectively. The personnel are simply not ready.

The third factor that has made it difficult for the industry to expand its range of services is the inflexible character of the regulations by which the industry is governed. The regulations provide little if any funding and almost no incentive for the industry to develop new programs. They are totally biased against the proprietary sector, and they do little to encourage the voluntary sector to become involved.

We must overcome these problems through a sustained effort to educate society as to what is happening now, rather than 10 to 20 years ago. We need to plan better for the future and to come to terms with the mistakes of the past: lack of funding, lack of training, lack of research, lack of resources, and promises of utopia by politicians.

The public should be better informed about the needs and characteristics of the elderly, those inside and those outside nursing facilities. The average income of the elderly is less than $2,000 a year, and the average age of the population in long-term care facilities is about 78–80. Three of every four patients are women. The average patient has at least three or four chronic illnesses at any given time. Many have outlived their families or friends. Approximately 65 percent of the patients in long-term care facilities are subsidized by a federal and state program. (This percentage will increase in the near future.) Some people in long-term care facilities could go home or to another living environment, but they would subsidies to do so. On the other hand, there are many who need care who are waiting to get into facilities. These people often require a comprehensive program of services.

It is my feeling that no one sector can solve the problems of the elderly and handicapped in our society. There will have to be a cooperative effort made by all. The long-term care industry can play an important part in finding solutions, but it can do this only if there is a change in the approach of Congress, regulatory agencies, and the consumer advocates. It is the responsibility of the leaders in every walk of life to stop using long-term

care facilities as the whipping boy for failures of society. With the cooperation of the government and the public, we could help provide a decent life
for many needy senior and handicapped citizens.

CHANGES IN THE SYSTEM

There are many problems with the regulatory processes affecting our
institutions. I would like to isolate some problems that appear particularly
significant to the administrator of a long-term care facility and to provide
suggestions for changes in the system. Many of these suggestions have, of
course, been made before, and some changes are in process even now.

As a general rule, our government officials at every level have a
tendency to impose regulatory solutions to all public problems brought to
their attention. In my opinion, this continual recourse to regulation has led
to an adversary situation in which the consumer is pitted against the
institution and the institution against the government. The industry finds
itself encumbered with stifling rules and regulations and forced to operate
in an atmosphere of contention and distrust. In order to correct this
adversary situation, some system should be developed whereby government and industry sit down together when a problem arises and make an
effort to work out the problem before regulation is invoked. Such a system
requires a sense of respect, of credence, and of acceptance on the part of all
parties. It places a responsibility on all of us to educate ourselves about the
consequences of legislation for all parties concerned. We must develop the
ability to forecast the real benefits and detriments of legislation as quickly
as possible and to plan the system to adjust to inequities rapidly. We must
acknowledge that there are no satisfactory legislative solutions to all problems, and that in some cases, legislation should give way to conditions
within the marketplace.

A long period of time is required for legislation to be conceived,
passed, interpreted as a set of regulations, and implemented. In many cases
the industry responds on a voluntary basis to public opinion and corrects a
problem before regulations are finalized. In other cases, legislation solves
the problem in theory but not in actual practice. We must create a system
whereby decision makers are kept apprised of developments in the industry as they occur.

The industry cannot expect an end to regulation; we will always be
regulated and controlled as long as the government is footing the bill. We
recognize also that the system must take over if voluntary solutions cannot
be found. Nevertheless, I believe that it is possible to improve the system
of regulation and to promote greater exchange between government, industry, and the public in the matter of long-term care.

One step which should be taken to achieve these objectives is the creation of a cabinet post to deal with the health and social health needs of the elderly and chronically ill. The individual chosen for the post would oversee and coordinate the administration of the various programs which presently serve the aged population. A more centralized system of authority might bring about an end to duplication and waste in these programs. This official might also authorize research to identify and interpret the needs of the target population in relation to the population as a whole. Finally, he would be charged with creating a system for the allocation and development of the resources necessary to accomplish these goals.

I propose also that studies be undertaken to determine the cost impact of regulatory measures. If the industry does not have sufficient funds to implement these measures, then some plan for resource development should be initiated. The regulatory agency should field-test regulations whenever possible and allow a reasonable period of time for industry to comply with any measure which proves to necessitate drastic changes. The "comments period," during which regulations can be discussed and questioned, should also be extended.

There should be greater flexibility in the enforcement of regulations. Federal regulations must be interpreted in accordance with local standards of acceptance. When national codes are formulated as regulations, government must be attentive to the effects of these codes on present structures and be willing to consider alternative solutions. Long-term care administrators who have expertise in the delivery of care should play an important role in the development and implementation of regulatory measures. Enforcement agencies must be better organized and employ better qualified and trained surveyors. The concept of enforcement itself should be modified: presently regarded as a punitive process, it should be approached instead as a form of education and improvement. As a final recommendation, I would suggest that incentives be built into the regulatory mechanisms to insure the effective delivery of services.

In my opinion, no foolproof system of regulatory control can ever be developed. It is particularly unfortunate, however, that regulations and legislation in the long-term care sector have been enacted in an atmosphere of hysteria and emotionalism unmatched in any other sector of the health care field. I recognize that the problems have existed and continue to exist, and that government concern was and is necessary. But it is unfair that the industry be made the scapegoat. It is now time to eliminate politics and emotionalism from our approach to long-term care problems. Perhaps we can start looking ahead to the development of a constructive and meaningful program for our elderly and chronically ill. Government cannot do it alone. Society cannot do it alone. The industry cannot do it alone—we must do it together.

8

COST IMPACT OF FEDERAL REGULATIONS
AND STANDARDS FOR NURSING HOMES

Harvey Carmel

This chapter treats the cost impact of federal regulations on nursing homes under Titles 18 and 19 of the Social Security Act. The discussion of this subject will be carried out at the micro level; it will center, in other words, on the effect of the regulations on the individual institution. The nature of individual responses to the regulatory process and standards will then be taken as a basis to make some general comments on the cost impact of regulations on the nursing home industry and the health care system in general.

It is my contention that all proposed regulations should be subjected to a cost impact analysis before they are submitted to the legislature. The cost assessments would serve a purpose similar to that served by environmental impact statements in other federal programs. Although certain cost estimates for nursing home regulations are required at present, they are neither useful nor adequate; they are made during the legislative process and they are typically concerned with program costs as opposed to system costs.[1] The economic costs of regulations exceed those incurred by the institution or program and include the spillovers into other areas of the health care marketplace and into the economy in general.

In order to develop a framework for the evaluation of the economic consequences of regulation, some understanding of the nature of costs in nursing homes is necessary. The chapter begins with an examination of the costs of operating a nursing home and moves to a consideration of the costs of coming to, and operating at, full compliance with the existing federal regulations. Once these costs are assessed, the chapter takes up the implications of cost impact on the regulatory process.

The basis for this paper and the evaluative framework presented is a model developed to estimate the cost impact of the 1974 federal regulations on SNFs and ICFs and a test application of it in the state of Minnesota.

OPERATING COSTS

Nursing home operating costs, and, in particular, costs per patient day (ppd), vary from one facility to the next. The data which follow should be viewed with this variation in mind; the operating costs have been averaged over all facilities surveyed. The factors that influence cost include the scope of services provided; the utilization rate; the age, location, and construction type of the facility; and the degree of compliance with regulations. Patient mix is a factor as well; the greater the percentage of complex cases, the greater the institutional costs. The relationship of facility size to cost is not yet clear, but the average cost ppd is observed to increase with increasing size. Other factors, however, might account for, or at least contribute to, such a relationship: larger facilities may offer more and different services, and/or have a higher percentage of complex cases than small ones. Finally, ownership may have a significant effect on costs. The 1973 Nursing Home Survey showed costs ppd for nonprofit homes to be greater than for proprietary homes. At a minimum, return on equity for proprietary homes affects cost. This difference may also be influenced by factors such as institutional philosophy, management techniques, patient selection, and type and quality of services rendered.

Costs themselves fall into the traditional classification of fixed and variable, where the variable costs are a function of the volume of services. The general types of expenses experienced by institutions are salaries and benefits for manpower, capital expenditures for physical plant or equipment for operating purposes, equipment maintenance, and overhead costs for heat, light, power, taxes, and so forth. Depreciation costs are considered independently of general overhead since regulations on nursing homes frequently relate to physical plant requirements, which are manifested as program costs in the form of depreciation. "Money costs" (such as interest expenses and return on equity) should also be included in expenditures.

An analysis of the existing federal regulations and the nature of nursing homes' operations identified 13 cost centers as the major units for apportioning operating costs. These cost centers are: nursing services, dietary services, diagnostic services, therapy services, recreational services, medical records, administrative services, laundry, housekeeping, pharmacy, utilization review and professional services, plant operation, and other expenses. For specific modeling purposes these cost centers may

have to be modified in order to reflect the data availability and the nature of
the regulations being studied. For example, they were modified in the
Minnesota study in order to reflect the nature of data available. In developing the cost estimation model for the SNF and ICF regulations, a detailed
chart of accounts was developed based upon the estimated sensitivity and
nature of costs attributable to the regulations in each cost center. This chart
allows the analyst to model the exact nature of the cost impact and to
isolate costs as completely as possible.

The general proportion of facility costs by cost center may be illustrated by the results of the Minnesota case study. Some of the major cost
centers and the percentage of the total cost they represented, measured at
actual level of compliance for 1975 for SNFs, were:

Nursing services	37.7
Dietary	16.0
Laundry, plant, housekeeping	12.5
Property (including depreciation, taxes)	9.9
Benefits	8.1
Administration	7.0

In contrast to:

Utilization review and professional services	1.6
Recreational activity	1.5
Other care and social services	1.7
Total salaries	65.9
Total consultant fees	1.9

The rank order of the relative percentage of contribution to costs by cost
centers for ICFs was not substantially different from the rank order for
SNFs.

The distribution of costs and the relative importance of each cost
center are significant. Consider the government regulation that impacts on
a cost center claiming a high percentage of the total costs of a nursing home.
Even a small change in that cost center may result in a very significant
change in cost to the institution. The converse is also true, so that a large
percentage change in a cost center that represents a modest share of the
total expenses will not have as great an absolute significance.

THE COSTS OF COMING TO FULL COMPLIANCE
WITH EXISTING FEDERAL REGULATIONS

The application of the Standards Impact Model is an example of an approach to analyzing regulations for cost impacts. This section is based again upon the case study in Minnesota. There was no attempt to assess the impacts for other states or for the United States in general since this was outside the scope of the study. It would be difficult to make any extensions since the cost impact is to a large degree a function of the location, state regulations, and the inspection process.

Before describing the findings, I would like to make a few general comments on the techniques and problems of estimating cost and the study process for the model. It is, after all, the framework which is the most important consideration. The model was developed from an analysis of each regulation in the federal SNF and ICF regulations. The nature of the cost impact and cost centers affected were isolated for each regulation. The amount of impact was estimated and only those centers for which a potential measurable expense was predicted were modeled.

Let us consider two specific examples and the techniques for estimating their costs. One of the most direct standards and easiest to model is the standard relating to the requirement for registered nurses, director of nursing (DON), and charge nurses on each shift for SNFs. The cost center affected by the regulation is Nursing Services; the nature of the impact concerns wages and benefits. The cost of compliance is then measured as the difference between the projected salaries at the minimum staffing level and the actual average staffing costs observed in facilities. Because of the intrafacility cost variance, facilities should be partitioned, that is, classified on the basis of the attributes so that they can be grouped as homogeneously as possible in order to account for as much of the intrainstitutional cost variances as possible. The specific partitioning for each cost center varied with the nature of the costs being studied. For example, costs associated with nursing salaries are sensitive to both facility size and location (urban or rural) and facility ownership, while certain physical plant expenditures, such as the cost of sprinkling systems, may be sensitive to location only.

As a second and more complex example, let us consider the standards for medical records in SNFs. The standards relate to personnel who have responsibility for records and to record storage, access, and content requirements. The content requirements that may have the most significant impact are those which dictate that each patient record include a treatment plan, assessment of patient's needs, record of services provided, diagnosis, report of physical and history, progress notes and observations, and report of treatments and clinical findings. The first order and immediate impact is in the medical records cost center as wages and benefits for the

medical records personnel and as depreciation for physical plant requirements for records storage and processing. While physical plant requirements represent immediate cost they are recaptured by institutions as
depreciation. There are also second order effects on nursing, administrative, and physician services. These effects are manifested as personnel
time required to meet content requirements. The second order effects are
costs to the homes or the patient directly (that is, reflected in charges for the
physician's time and visits). Nursing homes indirectly meet the content
requirements by adjusting their staffing pattern, or passing the costs on to
the program from which the administrative costs are incurred or to the
patient himself. In those cases where the individual physician is responsible for completing the record, he will generally figure his time in his
charges to the patient. The point to be made here is that each regulation
must be examined to determine whether there are effects beyond the first
order impact where one might expect to find the principal cost impact.

The process of modeling costs is not always straightforward. Regulations can be interpreted differently—by the provider who must comply
with them, the surveyor who must ascertain whether they have been met,
or the researcher who wishes to estimate the costs of coming to full
compliance with them. Consider, for example, the standards that specify
that services "adequate to meet the needs of patients" must be provided or
the regulatory provisions that are subject to waiver "if there is no impact on
the safety and health of patients." The language of the regulations raises a
new set of problems: the problems of determining what level of services is
"adequate," or of singling out those measures that will jeopardize the
safety and health of patients. Particular standards that rely for their interpretation on the judgment of the individual include those which call for
adequate nursing services (beyond the DON and charge nurse), for consultant dietetic services of sufficient duration and frequency, and for adequate social service facilities. In constructing our model, the problem
confronting us most directly was that of quantifying such concepts as
"adequacy" and "sufficiency." We consulted a panel of experts in nursing
home operations who were familiar with local problems and patient load.
With their assistance, we were able to impute any missing values by
applying a nominal group method (the Delphi Technique). An alternative
approach would be to impute values from those facilities historically recognized as certified to be in compliance.

In the Minnesota study, the cost impact of compliance was measured
against the baseline status of facilities in November 1975. The major impact
of federal regulations has probably already been experienced because the
Social Security Act was passed in 1965. However, there has been a liberal
granting of waivers and a general laxity of enforcement in some states. It
was hypothesized that there existed a substantial number of facilities still

TABLE 8.1

Total Annual Marginal Cost Impact of Full Compliance with Federal Regulations in Minnesota Nursing Homes as of November 1975

	Annual Individual Facility	Per Patient Day	Aggregate State	Number of Facilities
All SNFs	$32,923	$1.40	$8,098,964	246
All ICF-Is	$26,143	$1.17	$7,635,304	292
All ICF-IIs	$9,866	$1.52	$1,361,543	138

Source: Final Report: Assessment of Cost and Operational Impacts of SNF/ICF Standards, Vol. II., Oper., SRS, DHEW, JWK International Corp., Annandale, Virginia. July 27, 1976, Sec. I-9.

not in full compliance as required by P.L. 92-603. If the hypothesis were true, then there would have been a real cost impact measured if full compliance were required. This hypothesis, in fact, was substantiated by the Minnesota study.

The study findings were that full compliance of the federal regulations in Minnesota would result in increasing average annual facility expenditures in 1975 on the order of 5 percent for SNFs, 8 percent for ICF-Is, and 6 percent for ICF-IIs. Table 8.1 presents the marginal cost of compliance in dollar amounts.

While the cost impact per facility appears to be small, the cumulative effect of full compliance in the state is significant. The total annual increase over the 1975 level of costs if all SNFs and ICFs were operating at full compliance would be on the order of $17 million. The cost would be distributed among private pay, Medicaid, Medicare, and other public and private programs. Federal intervention here in a limited portion of the marketplace has spill-over effects to the nonfederal programs and to the entire industry by virtue of the fact that costs are increased for nonfederal payers through developing federal regulations. One group that would be affected by increased costs are the private insurance companies that have clients in long-term care institutions. Although these companies do not now contribute significantly to the financing of long-term care, they would eventually absorb some of the costs of full compliance. Also there may be a substantial cost impact on self-paying long-term care residents.

As mentioned above, facility costs vary with many factors. An analysis of the costs by homogeneous partitions showed that the percentage increase in annual facility costs for compliance ranged from 3 percent to 9 percent for SNFs, from 5 percent to 10 percent for ICF-Is, and from 3 percent to 7 percent for ICF-IIs. There was a larger percent of increases for rural facilities for both SNFs and ICFs than for urban ones. For example, urban SNFs would have a 4 percent increase, as opposed to a 9 percent increase for rural SNFs. This variation perhaps can be attributed to wage differences and the availability of such medical resources as trained personnel and supplies; however, there may be other influences such as services, patient load, and occupancy rates. Further research is necessary to isolate the causes. We might conclude from these findings that standards may need to vary by geography to reflect the availability and cost of medical resources. (Outside evaluation surveys at a subsequent time may show that standards can vary and that there is insufficient reason to hold both rural and urban facilities to the same input-based standards.) Furthermore, we might argue that reimbursement systems must allow for the geographic cost differences, particularly if incentive systems are to be developed.

Nonprofit SNFs and ICF-Is were estimated to have a greater cost increase than proprietary homes. The converse was true for ICF-IIs; proprietary ICF-IIs would experience a greater cost impact than their nonprofit counterparts. No clear conclusion could be drawn with respect to difference by size and governmental stature.

The analysis of compliance impact by cost center showed that the three centers with the largest dollar impact were nursing services, medical records, and recreational activities. When we restated the cost impacts as a percentage increase in costs over the 1975 costs or as a percentage of total marginal impact cost, we found that our hypothesis, that the largest impact would come from salaries and benefits for SNFs, was substantiated. For SNFs there was a 7 percent increase in salaries and benefits that accounted for 91 percent of the total impact. The case was similar for ICF-Is (10 percent increases and 99 percent of impact) and ICF-IIs (8 percent increases and 99 percent of impact).

There was a large dollar contribution to cost increases from nursing services. This is a case where a cost center that accounts for a large portion of facility costs (37.7 percent) would have a relatively small percentage increase in costs for compliance (6 percent) but a significant absolute dollar impact at compliance. In fact, the nursing services cost center in SNFs accounted for 40 percent of the total cost increases. Conversely, for small cost centers, even large percentage impacts had a small total dollar impact. Medical records in SNFs, which had the largest percent increase in costs (257 percent), accounted for only 26 percent of the total increase on a facility basis.

The cost center impacts also varied by facility attributes. Although the variations observed did not, in general, fall into any special patterns, cost impacts were estimated to be generally higher for rural facilities. For example, the nursing service impact for rural SNFs was 11 percent, while the impact for urban SNFs was only 3 percent. Similarly, recreation activities impact for urban ICF-Is was 14 percent, but for rural facilities, 215 percent.

My purpose in undertaking an investigation of this kind was to demonstrate the usefulness of an impact estimation system. Such a system would enable us to test the impact of proposed regulations before they were actually put into effect and to determine whether the demands we sought to place on individual facilities were, in fact, realistic ones. Therefore, in the course of the project, we examined more than 30 individual regulations to determine their impacts on full compliance costs. The greatest impact arose from the Minnesota state requirement that each patient in an SNF or ICF-I receive two hours of nursing care each day and from the state recommendation that the activities staff allot two thirds of an hour each day to each patient. These two Minnesota regulations, together with the federal regulation on medical records, accounted for 81 percent of the total SNF impact. The requirements for a medical director, a charge nurse, and dietetic services accounted for the remaining 19 percent of SNF impact.

The model structure applied state standards where they existed and exceeded federal ones or in those cases where federal regulations were not quantified. The use of state standards is valid since federal regulation requires state licensure and conformity with all state standards. In addition, these state standards can be viewed as acceptable minimum levels where federal regulations are silent or not quantified.

As part of the Minnesota investigation, we performed some sensitivity studies to assess the impact that various modifications of the standards would have on facility costs. For example, we increased the nursing coverage requirements to around-the-clock RN services in SNFs. This change resulted in an almost 23 percent increase in the impact and a 1.2 percent increase in the total annual cost above that already measured to come to full compliance. When we increased SNF medical director requirements to 8 hours each week, we found an 8.4 percent change in the impact and a four-tenths of a percent increase in total annual costs. One modification that had a particularly significant effect involved the requirement for records clerks. If we decreased that requirement by changing the imputed value of one clerk for each 50 patients to 1 for each 60 patients, it resulted in a 14.4 percent decrease of the impact and a 0.8 percent decrease in operating costs.

The approach to date has been to estimate the costs of legislation or regulation at the program or the sponsoring agency level. There has been little attention paid to the impact on the individual institution and its ability to absorb the changes. Moreover, the macro-level impact on the health system has also been overlooked. The macro-level impact may manifest itself as increased costs to other payors and society, and as changes in the availability, accessibility, and "quality" of services rendered. In evaluating the macro-level impact, we must consider more than just the sum of the individual institutional responses; we should recognize the spill-over of the costs of regulation into other areas of the health sector and the economy in general—for example, in the form of inflationary pressure.

Individual nursing homes can respond to regulations by passing costs on to the program, passing excess or nonreimbursable costs on to the patient, changing the nature and quantity of services, electing not to participate in the program, or discontinuing services altogether. From the program perspective, the sum of the individual responses constitutes the total impact on the program. However, macro-impacts are not equal to the sum of individual costs. For example, a requirement for additional nursing services may increase demand drastically and possibly result in an upward pressure on wages, which could carry over to the hospital sector as well. Likewise, regulations may be biased toward institutionalization and result in disincentives to develop alternative sources and types of care. Regulators tend to take the perspectives of their own program and regulatory agency and to ignore other perspectives and alternative ways of reaching the desired results. If costs are not matched to reimbursement and if institutions do not have sufficient revenue after meeting expenses to absorb the extra cost (or the option of passing these costs on to patients), then the institutions may elect to withdraw from the program or cease operation totally. We might then find a shrinkage in the supply of providers.

In Minnesota for example, from September 1973 to June 1976, the supply of SNFs increased by 9 percent; however, the number of ICFs dropped by 22 percent. Nineteen percent of the drop occurred within six months of the implementation (January 1975) of the current regulations, while 2 percent occurred between August 1975 and February 1976. Most of those who withdrew from Medicaid were ICF-IIs, and some of those who withdrew are now participating in SSI. There is no evidence yet of a trend toward nonprofit or proprietary institutions or toward larger institutions as a result of these regulations. Likewise, while the change in numbers of providers was uniform over rural and urban providers, this trend must be monitored since the cost impact for full compliance is greater on rural homes than on urban homes. A geographic maldistribution of facilities could develop if the cost differentials are not incorporated into the reimbursement system.

The introduction of a cost-estimating technique would be the necessary first step in an effort to relate the activities of regulation and reimbursement. Other writers have argued that one agency should be responsible for the establishment of reimbursement rates and the inspection of facilities (an inspection carried out to determine whether individual institutions are complying with regulatory standards). I would extend their argument by calling for some type of formal cooperation between the individuals who establish the rates and the individuals who actually devise the regulatory standards. At present, the communication between the agencies that perform these functions is notoriously poor. We have one arm of the government developing regulations that increase costs and another arm of the government refusing to make accommodations for these increases in costs. While the division of responsibility may not be a major impediment to a national system under Medicare, which has a cost-based reimbursement plan, it does pose considerable difficulties for the Medicaid program. We need, then, to direct our efforts toward the creation of a reimbursement policy that is sensitive to the changes in regulatory standards and to the cost impact of those changes on the long-term care institutions. Likewise, the maximum benefits of such cost estimation techniques cannot be realized fully until a quality measurement system is developed relating facility standards to patient needs and outcomes. A cost/benefit analysis of alternative regulations requires that there exist a method to compare output measures of regulations and their contribution to reaching a desired objective. Currently, regulations are generally stated on an input basis without any clear understanding of their impact on, and relationship to, patient outcomes.

The language and format of the regulations may also have certain cost implications that merit our attention. We have seen that some regulations are formulated in nonquantifiable terms and are subject to the interpretation of the survey and the researcher alike. While the lack of quantification is not in itself a serious indictment of the regulatory process, it is evident that we cannot expect survey teams to make normative judgments on a scientific and objective basis about the adequacy of a service. The problem is compounded by the fact that we have no reliable methods for evaluating the quality of care of predicting the relationships between inputs and patient outcomes. We have, in my opinion, an anomalous situation where the regulations and process are more advanced—that is, in the sense of being flexible and related to patient assessment and needs—than the state of the arts of standard making and quality evaluation necessary to support the regulations constructed in this fashion. If operative systems for measuring outcome and assessing patient needs existed, then the use of flexible regulations would be desirable. Institutions would then have the discretionary powers to meet the needs of their patients and to assure consistency of outcomes, at the same time they would be able to allocate costs internally in the most effective manner. This flexibility and the quality measures based on patient assessment status could then be tied into some incentive reimbursement system in order to help control costs. As a short term solution, however, quantifiable guidelines that do not have the effect of regulation would help surveyors reduce variance in their interpretations of the regulations.

So that policymakers might have a more accurate understanding of the impact of regulation on institutions, some attention should also be given to the present system of data collection. In the past, we have lacked a sufficient data base by which to measure regulatory impact. For example, even though our model was sensitive enough to measure the cost impact of Life Safety Code compliance and the second order and perhaps real cost impact of staff development, we could not, in fact, determine these costs because the necessary data were not available. Improvements in the system might, of course, prove costly to the institutions; the extensive sight surveys and paperwork that data collection generally entails could impose additional administrative costs upon the provider. In the long run, however, the information gathered would give government policymakers a better sense of the economics of the provider's position. The trade-offs must be considered, but it is my feeling that some revision of the information system is necessary to the development of a rational regulatory policy.

NOTE

1. This chapter, in fact, is based upon a model that was developed to estimate the cost of the 1974 Regulations of SNFs and ICFs. The project was funded by the Department of Health, Education, and Welfare; significantly, it was funded after the regulations were promulgated.

A more detailed presentation of the model can be found in the reports to the Department of Health, Education, and Welfare: *Development of a Model to Estimate Cost of Compliance with SNF and ICF Standards*, March 3, 1975, for BQA, HSA, DHEW, Contract No. HSM 110-73-500, Applied Management Sciences, Silver Spring, Md.; and *Assessment of Cost and Operational Impacts of SNF/ICF Standards*, April 23, 1976, for SRS, HSA, DHEW, SRS-500-75-0032, by JWK International Corp., Annandale, Virginia.

9
CAPITAL AND THE REIMBURSEMENT OF
THE COSTS OF NURSING HOME SERVICES *

Kenneth M. McCaffree
Suresh Malhotra
John Wills

ISSUES IN CAPITAL REIMBURSEMENT

A major issue in the reimbursement of the costs of nursing home services under the Medicaid program has been the determination of the rent for capital resources.† In recent years, no aspect of nursing home care reimbursement has received more attention, nor has any created more public debate. Nursing home owners and administrators, claiming inadequate profits, have asked for increased rates of property cost reimbursement. They have demanded specific regulations under Section 249 of PL 92-603, which would allow the states to include a profit factor in a cost-related reimbursement system. Some public officials and citizen groups have been critical of large capital gains that resulted from the sale and resale of facilities during recent periods of rapid inflation and substantially increased demand for nursing home services. Medicaid officials have voiced concern about increased annual depreciation costs, the result of higher purchase prices for nursing homes. Charges of a "rip-off" have frequently been leveled against the nursing home industry because rent levels in some cases have been increased by sale-lease back arrangements

*The authors acknowledge that part of the effort in the preparation of this chapter was supported by Contract No. 600-77-0069 to the Battelle Human Affairs Research Centers from the Office of Policy Planning and Research, Health Care Financing Administration, U.S. Department of Health, Education, and Welfare.
†"Rent" or "rents" for capital resources are used to parallel "wage" or "wages" for labor resources. We use "rents" in a general sense to include all components in the reimbursement for capital resources.

between affiliated organizations. These issues in capital reimbursement are largely unsettled and continue to be the subject of legal, political, and economic debate.

The primary purposes of this chapter are to consider several economic aspects of the capital reimbursement issue and to suggest principles that may help to solve some of the current problems in establishing rents for capital resources in nursing homes. In any regulated industry, the determination of rent levels poses certain problems, but in the case of the nursing home reimbursement system, it is complicated by the lack of clearly defined policy goals. Efforts to identify the objectives appropriate to a reimbursement system for nursing home care should be undertaken as part of the solution of the economic issues. In this section, we briefly consider the complexities inherent in capital reimbursement and also suggest some criteria for the consideration of alternative capital reimbursement schemes. In the next section, the practice of "trafficking" in nursing homes is used to illustrate the capital reimbursement issues specific to determining rent levels in a reimbursement system for nursing home care. The final section sets forth alternative plans for setting rent on capital resources in nursing homes.

Complexities in Determining Rents

The complexities involved in determining proper reimbursement for capital assets are readily apparent when we compare capital resource payments with compensation of labor services. In the case of labor, wages are for the most part directly observable from reasonably well-established labor markets, and the transactions between employer and employee are easily recorded in the accounts of the nursing home firm. Setting labor service prices is difficult only for self-employed and unpaid family workers. Wage rates for the services of these people, however, can be determined by observing market rates of pay for comparable workers.

The services of capital assets may also be purchased in the market directly or obtained from assets owned by the firm. The services of the capital stock, like those of labor, must be compensated. However, no clear-cut measures of opportunity costs are available because there are no well-established markets for the services of specific capital. The rent of firm-owned capital is therefore especially difficult to determine. Furthermore, because capital assets can be bought and sold whereas workers cannot, numerous financing arrangements for obtaining capital services are possible and may further complicate efforts to determine the market cost of the services provided. Assets may be leased, owned outright by the firm, or obtained by a combination of leasing, owning or financing through borrowed funds used to purchase the assets. These capital asset contracts are usually long term and are set out in dollar terms rather than in terms of real goods and services in the accounting records of the firm. Changes in the dollar will therefore cause accounting values to diverge from market values. In addition to these factors, capital assets, unlike labor, are exhausted in the production process. This use of capital, routinely referred to as depreciation, represents an expense or cost to be covered by the revenue earned by the firm. The extent to which the amount of depreciation recorded in the accounts of the firm differs from true economic depreciation further complicates how rent for capital resources is handled. Finally, the measurement of a premium for the risk assumed by the owner/entrepreneur increases the difficulties in fixing a rent for capital in a cost-related reimbursement system. The residual between total revenues and total expenditures has been associated with entrepreneurship and owner/operator capital. Since this residual may be negiative or positive, the owner/entrepreneur assumes a risk that other participants in the firm, including workers, do not. Consequently, he will require compensation in relation to the risk burden undertaken. No very effective means has been developed for determining the risk premium in rent payments.

Criteria for Rate-Setting Policy

Although the major problem considered in this chapter is how to overcome the complexities of capital resource reimbursement in order to set a price or reimbursement rate for nursing home services, the identification and definition of criteria for rate-setting and reimbursement policy are necessary. In order to proceed on a clear basis of understanding and to avoid an extended discussion of alternative criteria, we first suggest some economic and policy standards against which to measure the effectiveness of alternative capital reimbursement schemes. In addition, we summarize those characteristics of the nursing home industry that have some relevance for the selection of a reimbursement plan and for the determination of rents for capital resources.

Policy Norms

The "product" of health services and nursing home care must be defined before we can establish norms for rate setting. Although our definition is not entirely satisfactory, we propose that the product be called a "standard patient day." This is analogous to the use of homogeneous units of labor time in labor market analyses.

The economic efficiency of a reimbursement system is a major consideration. In an efficient system, a group of facilities with similar economic characteristics and opportunities produce nursing home services at
a minimum average cost for each unit of product. Unless otherwise justified, each facility's production should be regulated so that average cost for
each unit of product is at a minimum. If this criterion is to be applied,
however, the regulators must provide some assurance that product quality
will be maintained. In the absence of well-defined outcomes of care, we
propose that the quality of nursing home care should be no less than that
which satisfies professional standards of inputs and processes of care.

Another issue that merits consideration is how the reimbursement
system affects various types of organizations. Under a given reimbursement system, will profit-making nursing homes fare better than voluntary
nursing homes, or will sole proprietorships fare better than multifacility
national nursing home firms? Any rate-setting methodology favoring one
type over another should be justified in terms of variations in quality of
nursing home care and minimum average costs for each unit of output. In
addition, the reimbursement rate should be neutral with respect to incentives for the expansion or contraction of the industry's capacity. In the
absence of a policy to expand capacity, the payment to owners of capital
resources, as the risk takers in the industry, should be set so that there is no
desire either to increase or to decrease the quantity of capital invested in
the industry, relative to alternative investment opportunities.*

Industry Characteristics

In designing a reimbursement plan and establishing rents for capital
resources, government must take into account certain characteristics of
the nursing home industry. The industry is primarily proprietary, con-
sisting for the most part of small firms. It is basically competitive, with new
firms able to enter the system with ease, except as entry is limited by
certificate-of-need legislation and licensing regulations.

Government is the major purchaser of the industry product. It
possesses actual (potential) monopsonistic market power, which generally
manifests itself in quality of care specifications and regulations rather than
in the price of nursing homes per se. The government's role as regulator in

---

*Another broad policy alternative could be introduced at this point, namely whether or
not to regulate the nursing home industry. Although we consider this issue briefly below,
regulation and its associated real costs must be less than the marginal social benefits obtained
in regulating the industry, a fact that to our knowledge has yet to be established.

this case is due to its function as a major purchaser and is not due to anticompetitive activities of the industry. Government regulation does not imply that competition cannot exist among nursing homes.

A large number of consumers are mentally or physically handicapped and are unable to compare alternative suppliers and products in order to select the most advantageous benefit/price relationship. Other consumers are poor and unable to purchase essential nursing home services. In the latter case, government agencies, using public funds, act as purchasers and third-party payers.

ISSUES IN SETTING RENTS
IN THE NURSING HOME INDUSTRY

The principal issues in the determination of appropriate rents for capital resources in the nursing home industry have been highlighted by the frequent sale and resale of facilities. This practice of "trafficking" in nursing homes usually takes the form of the sale of facilities by one firm to its fully owned subsidiaries or "dummy" corporations.

Several regulatory agencies and government investigative groups have been studying the problem of trafficking in recent years. The staff of the New York State Moreland Act Commission developed simulation models to determine the potential consequences of trafficking. The results of these simulations, based on the discounted cash flow method of estimating rates of return, showed annual rates of return on initial investments of nearly 30 percent over short periods of time.[1] Although the actual extent to which homes were sold and resold, to our knowledge, has yet to be tabulated in any systematic fashion, the reactions to large potential gains were sufficient to prompt a U.S. Department of Health, Education, and Welfare reimbursement proposal that allowed no payment for the services of operator-owned capital resources.* The Moreland Act Commission recommended a fixed long-term "fair rental" return in which the nursing home assets were treated essentially as bonds. Certificate-of-need legislation was passed in several states in an attempt to reduce sales, and additional regulations and restrictions were drawn up to specify the conditions under which nursing homes could be sold, rented, or placed under new management.

---

*One of the early drafts of regulations under Section 249 of P.L. 92-603 excluded any payment for the services of equity capital.

Our discussion of trafficking and capital reimbursement issues is divided into three parts. The first is an analysis of the components in the reimbursement of capital. The second part is a brief description of the method by which rents were determined under the state Medicaid reimbursement systems over the past few years. The conditions under which the sale and resale of nursing homes take place are discussed in the final part of this section.

Components in the Reimbursement for Capital Resources

Four components in the reimbursement of capital require definition and explanation for this discussion. These are: rent payments in owner wage payments, depreciation expense, the cost for capital services, and profits (or losses).*

Rents for capital resources may be included in the wage payments to an owner or to those members of a family who own and manage a nursing home. We see no major problems, however, in determining whether any payments to owner-contributed capital are included in family wage payments. These payments could be higher than market wages. However, estimating the market wage for labor services of the owner or other family members is rather straightforward. Wage rates for comparable jobs in other homes or businesses in the same community can usually be readily determined. Any difference between the total wage payments to owners and the going market wage for that type of labor service can be treated as if it were a payment for ownership of capital resources.

Depreciation is the extent to which an asset or capital stock is exhausted over some time period in the production process. Although most people are already familiar with this process (for example, they recognize that an automobile wears out as it is driven), the problems of evaluating the asset's depreciation in a given period and of determining whether this value is accurately reflected in the accounting records of the firm remain. The real market value and depreciation rate of an asset often differ from those recorded in the accounts. Discrepancies of this kind represent the chief

---

*We might have examined maintenance costs of property and capital assets here as well, but we have chosen to set these aside as part of the analysis of operating costs. Two points, however, should be noted. First, older assets may require more maintenance than newer ones. Second, the useful age of an asset, and hence its real depreciation rate, can be influenced by the extent and amount of maintenance undertaken with respect to the asset. Accordingly, in the final analysis, payments to capital resources must be reconciled to and considered in relation to operating costs, including capital resource maintenance costs.

problem state agencies face in their efforts to set reimbursement allowances for depreciation expenses.

The real or market value of an asset at any point in time is the discounted value of the expected stream of service from that asset. Thus, the annual net real depreciation is the difference in the discounted values of the expected stream of service at the beginning and at the end of the year. Annual accounting depreciation, however, is the distribution of the historical or "book" value of the asset over some assumed life of that asset, and is independent of current market values and future expectations. Various methods of formulas, such as straight-line or sum-of-digits, have been devised to estimate how much of the book value of a capital asset is used up in the production process in each accounting period. Straight-line depreciation, for example, assumes that the historical value of the asset should decline an equal amount during each period of the expected life of the asset.

There are several reasons why real depreciation will differ from accounting depreciation. First, accounting conventions are such that recorded depreciation bears little resemblance to the decline in the value of the service flow of physical assets. There is no reason to expect that the value of the service flow from a given asset, such as a nursing home facility, declines precisely in accordance with any depreciation method. In fact, tax regulations promote rapid accounting depreciation by allowing accelerated depreciation techniques and by permitting use of artificially short asset-lifetime guides. Second, the market continually reevaluates assets based on current market conditions, even if the length of asset life were accurately estimated. Unexpected revisions of market expectations may cause assets to rise or decline in value, and the book value of assets and annual accounting depreciation will diverge from real values. Furthermore, during a period of inflation, book accounts lose meaning rapidly as the market value of assets rises with the prices of all goods and services. The divergence of real depreciation from book depreciation is also related to the age of the asset since the purchase date. Finally, maintenance expenditures, recorded as operating expenses, may represent investments in increased asset durability. The fact that an owner/entrepreneur can *choose* the real depreciation rate is not even considered in accounting practices. In this case, the present value of the depreciation expenses allowed by the accounting method will exceed the present value of the real depreciation over the same period.

Capital cost is the payment for the services of capital, and is referred to as the return or interest on the invested capital. An observed return on an investment can be broadly defined to consist of a pure return to the use of the productive capital services and a return to the risk-bearing function of the capital owner. Risk is generally associated with uncertainty of earnings and is usually measured by the variability of the returns.

All resource use, of course, involves some risk to the owner.* Even though faced with some fluctuation in earnings, workers do have a prior claim to the revenues of the firm. Furthermore, expected variability in the earnings of capital and the claims on revenues will be different among those who provide capital because the financial or accounting forms of capital vary within and across firms. For example, the payments to capital resources contributed by an owner/entrepreneur of a nursing home (equity capital) are accorded only residual claim to the revenues of the firm. Debt capital resources are accorded prior claims to owner/entrepreneur capital. Where risk is measured by the variability in earnings over time, owner/entrepreneurs bear more risk than debt capital owners.

Thus, a major difficulty associated with the reimbursement of the cost of capital services is the allocation of the returns on capital to owners on the basis of risk sharing, as well as the productivity of the capital resources per se. Once debt capital in dollars has been transformed into real capital assets and owner capital in dollars has likewise taken the form of capital assets, the resources are indistinguishable. The productivity of capital resources financed by debt will not differ from the productivity of resources financed by owner/entrepreneur contributions. In other words, the contract between a lender and a borrower shifts some of the risk associated with a firms's use of capital resources to the borrower, who, for the assumption of such risk, claims some of the real value produced by the capital resources obtained by debt financing.

The accounting records of the firm, however, provide no direct insight into these issues. The cost of borrowed capital is recorded as an expenditure for interest. The net difference between revenues and expenditures on the books of the firm is profit and the payment for the services of equity capital. These book transactions are unlikely to equal the real return on capital resources. The basic reasons for this divergence are that accounting measures of net income do not correspond to the economic definition of income, and accounting measures of the capital stock diverge from market values as indicated in the section on depreciation expense.[2]

Whereas accounting profit is the net difference between recorded revenues and expenditures in a specific period, economic profit is the difference between the payment to a resource and what that resource would be paid in its most productive alternative use. Put another way, any

---

*Workers can expect some variability in relative wages over time, and in some cases face technological displacement and retraining costs in order to maintain an accustomed earnings level. Similarly, owners of capital resources are confronted with technological change and obsolescence, and the need to liquidate and reinvest in other opportunities.

payment or share of the firms's revenue received by a resource owner, in excess of what is necessary to induce that owner to employ that resource in the specific use, is "profit." It should be noted, of course, that residual revenues or payments, such as those made to nursing home owners for equity capital resources, may well be less than payments in alternative uses for the same capital. In this case, a "loss" is sustained even though the payment may, in fact, be greater than zero and the net income on the books of the firm is positive. At any one time, some capital owners in an industry may be making economic profits while others are incurring losses. In a perfectly functioning competitive market and in the absence of uncertainty, profit (or loss) would be zero in the long run.[3]

Determining Rents in State Reimbursement Systems

The determination of rents for capital resources has been an issue primarily in those states which have had cost-based reimbursement systems. Where nursing home services were paid for on a flat rate basis, only questions regarding excessive profits to owners have been seriously considered, and these were as much related to low quality of care as to capital reimbursement levels per se. Since 1972, when Congress mandated cost-related reimbursement for nursing home care under PL 92-603, states have been restructuring their reimbursement systems in order to comply with the statute and the HEW regulations that pertain to it. Most states now have some type of regulation or policy governing each of the components of capital reimbursement considered above.

Wages for owners and family members who work in the nursing home have generally been limited to the market wages of other workers supplying comparable services. Salary limits or limits on total allowed costs of administrative services are not uncommon. These regulations on administrative salaries have been used to avoid excessive wage and salary payment to sole proprietors, partners, and administrators of family-held corporations. Although precise data are not available, these regulations probably directly affect the salary and wage payments of owners in over half the firms in the industry.

State reimbursement systems have followed accounting practices exclusively in capital reimbursement regulations and have accordingly relied on book values. States have provided for straight-line depreciation, based on the historical cost of the asset, and including use of Internal Revenue Service guidelines for length of asset life. As late as 1974, three states used the original construction cost of the facility as the depreciation base. A few states have permitted an accelerated depreciation method for equipment when the method was accepted by the IRS. To our knowledge, no state has used replacement costs or a current appraised value of a facility as a base for annual depreciations, and no state has seriously considered major changes in the IRS depreciation guidelines on asset life.

The handling of capital costs has also followed conventional accounting practices. Interest payments on mortgages and borrowed funds were allowed, and only in the case of personal loans or notes by an owner to the nursing home were standards of "appropriate and reasonable" interest applied. Profit allowances for the services of the capital contributed by owners have been determined in several ways. Most states paid a rate of return on owner (equity) capital, based on historical or book values. Other states paid a fixed amount for each patient day or a fixed percent of certain allowed costs.

Finally, for most states a rent agreement between an owner and an administrator/operator was accepted and the rent allowed as contracted. In the last three or four years, regulations on "non-arm's length" rental transactions, such as those between a subsidiary and a parent corporation, or those between two organizations largely owned by the same individuals, have been extensively invoked. These rental agreements were subjected to "reasonableness" tests, and in some cases, capital was reimbursed as if the owner and operator companies were one and the same.

Table 9.1 summarizes the reimbursement practices in the state Medicaid programs for most of the above capital reimbursement components at the end of 1974. To our knowledge, no more recent detailed tabulation of these regulatory practices has been made.*

Conditions Encouraging Trafficking

Because the state reimbursement systems rely on certain accounting procedures in determining rents, they have failed to take into consideration the changes in market forces. Nevertheless, it is the divergence between the book and real values of assets that makes the sale and resale of nursing homes so attractive to owners—which creates, in short, the conditions conducive to "trafficking." When historical values diverge from market values, and reimbursement agencies ignore the discrepancy, owners of nursing home assets can usually increase real capital earnings by selling facilities or realigning ownership/leasing arrangements.

---

*We are aware from current research at the Battelle Health Care Study Center that changes have been occurring in the states, especially as flat-rate states have moved to cost-related reimbursement systems under P.L. 92-603; however, we have not systematically recorded these changes.

TABLE 9.1

Regulations on Rents in 36 State Reimbursement Systems, 1974*

Regulation	Number of States with Regulation
Administrative Salary Limits	13
Depreciation on Allowable Cost	36
Original Cost Depreciation Base Specified	3
Straight-line Depreciation Specified	19
Limits on Interest	4
Profits: Return on Equity	24
Payment Per Patient Day	7
Percent of Costs	5
Arms Length Transaction	14

*Only 36 states had cost-related reimbursement systems; Arizona and Alaska had no system, and the remaining 12 were states with flat-rate systems.

Source: K. M. McCaffree, et al. *Profits, Growth and Reimbursement Systems in the Nursing Home Industry.* Final Report to the Health Care Financing Administration under Conract No. 600-77-0069 to the Battelle Human Affairs Research Centers, Seattle, Washington (Forthcoming).

The sale of nursing homes generally takes place in one of two situations. First, facilities may be sold to increase the book value of capital. Historical costs (book values) in recent years have fallen substantially below the market value of nursing home assets. Since reimbursement for nursing home care has been based on book values of assets, owners have had an incentive to sell in order to raise the book value of nursing home assets upon which returns to equity capital are based. These gains raise the rents for nursing home capital to the going market rate on capital investments of comparable risk.* Under most reimbursement policies, mortgage interest payments have been covered carte blanche by the Medicaid reimbursement agencies. Thus, an owner could finance the purchase of a nursing home with a very small equity or down payment, hold the facility

---

*The difference in the sale price, which is measured in dollars that have depreciated in value because of inflation, and the dollar value of the initial (historical) investment could have been substantial. The real rate of return, measured in constant dollar terms, however, may well have been very close to real returns in other industries and investments.

for four years, collect the depreciation expense and full reimbursement of mortgage interest, and then sell the four-year-older facility in an inflationary economy at a higher price than was paid for it. The combination of depreciation expense, mortgage interest payment, and the gain in sale price over purchase price provides a much higher annual *real* rate of return on the small-owner equity investment than was allowed through the reimbursement system.

In the situation described, the substantial divergence of book and market values of assets and the character of the reimbursement policies clearly encouraged the practice of trafficking. As long as inflation continues and/or the demand for nursing home services increases relative to other goods and services, nursing homes will be sold and resold. Under existing reimbursement plans, investors will continue to seek this avenue to maximize real rates of return in nursing home investment.

The second situation in which the sale of a nursing home frequently takes place also reflects a divergence of market values and historical values. In this case, however, the "sale" occurs so that the present owner can continue operating the facility. This is the sale and lease-back arrangement in which the sale is generally made to an affiliated organization or wholly owned "dummy" corporation. Again, the purpose of such sale and lease arrangements is to bring depressed real rates of return in line with current market payments for capital resources.

Most Medicaid reimbursement systems allow for full rent when a facility is leased under an arm's-length transaction, which implies that the rent represents the going market rental price for these assets. The lease arrangement or the net rent typically includes the depreciation expense on a prospective and current market basis, and a current market-determined payment for the services of the assets. Since most lease contracts are short term and are frequently renegotiated annually, the lease or rent payments will be based on the current market value of the assets.

In the case of owner/entrepreneurs, depreciation expense and the payment for capital resource services are based on book and/or historical values under most state Medicaid reimbursement systems. Recognizing that an owner of a leased facility is receiving a current market level payment for the use of comparable assets, many owners have proceeded to divest themselves of their nursing home assets through sale and lease-back arrangements. In order to retain effective ownership, these owners have sold their facilities to a wholly owned subsidiary or similarly affiliated organization. They then argue for reimbursement of depreciation expense and payment for capital services based on market asset values—the type of arrangement found in an arm's-length rental contract.

Table 9.2 illustrates the two situations that have encouraged trafficking and sale-lease back arrangements in the nursing home industry. The divergence between market and book values of assets quickly results in a

TABLE 9.2

A Simulated Trend in Asset Values, Annual Depreciation, and Rents in Nursing Homes

Accounting Period (years)	Asset Value		Estimated Length of Asset Life[a] (years)	Annual Depreciation Allowance		Annual Cost of Capital Services (Estimated 10% of Asset Value)		Annual Total Rent	
	Market Value[a]	Book Value[a]		Market Value Base	Book Value Base	Value Base	Value Base	Market Value	Book Value
1	$100,000	$100,000	10	$10,000	$10,000	$10,000	$10,000	$20,000	$20,000
2	94,500[b]	90,000	9	10,500	10,000	9,450	9,000	19,950	19,000
3	88,000[b]	80,000	8	11,000	10,000	8,800	8,000	19,800	18,800
4	80,500[b]	70,000	7	Sells at $80,500		—	—	—	—
NEW OWNER									
1	80,500	80,500	7	11,500	11,500	8,050	8,050	19,550	19,500

aValues determined at the beginning of the year.
bA 5 percent annual increase in market value was assumed and added to the book value on the first day of each year.
Source: Compiled by the authors.

large difference in annual rents as well as capital gains, and provides an obvious reason for an owner to sell and for the purchaser to buy. In addition, owners who are reimbursed on historical values will obtain less annual rent for the same invested capital than will the owner who leases. Since the lease payment is based on current market values and is generally accepted as an allowed rental cost under conventional accounting and reimbursement practices, firms attempt to obtain the market rent by a sale and lease-back arrangement with an affiliated organization. In states where reimbursement regulations prohibit such sale and lease-back agreements, obvious differences in the reimbursement of capital resources arise between owner/operators on one hand and owner/lessors on the other.

ALTERNATIVE METHODS OF DETERMINING
CAPITAL REIMBURSEMENT

Trafficking in nursing homes is symptomatic of a larger problem. Reimbursement regulations conceived and carried out without regard to market adjustments produced by inflation, competition, and the normal search for profits clearly invite the sale and resale, or sale and lease-back, of facilities. Resource owners, whether worker or capitalist, owner/renter, or owner/operator of a nursing home, will seek that alternative employment, investment, or operating arrangement that at least assures each the going rate of payment for the productive capacity being offered. Regulations must, in our judgment, work with market forces, not against them, and must use the profit incentive and the avoidance of loss by all resource owners as the mechanism for achieving an efficient use of resources in the nursing home industry.[4] Hence, a reimbursement and regulatory scheme using these incentives effectively and working with market forces is most likely to realize the desired policy goals, and at the same time, to assure an efficient use of resources.*

We offer for consideration two alternatives for the reimbursement of capital resources. The first is a policy that relies on the market to set the price of nursing home services and that rewards capital owners in accordance with market activities. The second is a policy limited to the reimbursement of capital on the basis of a rental system. This second

---

*We recognize that policymakers, including taxpayers, may choose to create some economic inefficiency if necessary in order to achieve some other goal, such as equal geographic access to facilities or equal access to a given range of health services. We believe, however, that the wiser policy will result if the "cost" or "price" of the trade-off in terms of economic efficiency is known and understood.

approach allows for either an explicit or an implicit market rental system for the payment of capital resources under a cost-related reimbursement system. Each is briefly considered below.*

Nonregulation

Whether a policy of nonregulation can be made to work will depend upon the effectiveness of the market for nursing home services. The number of nursing homes is sufficient to assure a substantial measure of competition, and few of the 18,000 homes in the country are so isolated that they represent geographic monopolies. Collusion, of course, may occur. However, the costs of maintaining a cartel among even a small number of firms are great, and the short-run economic advantage a proprietary facility would gain by breaking away from the group might eventually threaten the stability of a cartel. Furthermore, active consumer protective organizations and the state and federal justice departments have repeatedly demonstrated their effectiveness in discouraging collusive behavior. Finally, the extensive development of alternatives to nursing homes, such as home health care agencies, visiting nurse services, meals on wheels, and other noninstitutional programs, would exert substantial competitive pressure on the nursing home industry.

The efficiency of the market may break down because of failures on the buying side rather than the lack of competition among nursing homes. Many individual purchasers are not able to appraise nursing home services and to make appropriate price comparisons among homes, and their misjudgments can result in an inefficient use of resources. Moreover, the failure of buyers in the private care market to assess the alternatives properly has not been corrected by the Medicaid agencies who have made extensive purchases of nursing home care; these agencies have frequently

---

*The statement of norms for rate setting and our discussion of the components of reimbursement for capital raise two issues that we do not discuss in the chapter. As a starting point in a policy for capital reimbursement, we propose that the difference between wage payments to owner/administrators (or family members) and earnings available from alternative employment opportunities should be included with payments to capital. Second, we do not analyze the conditions under which profit (or loss), as defined above, should be other than zero, that is, we do not examine the conditions under which the proper policy objective is to expand or to contract the capacity of the industry. We are concerned with the identification and determination of a rent for capital resources sufficient only to induce the owners of capital to invest that quantity of capital in nursing homes which simply maintains a given product capacity.

proven to be as undiscriminating as the private purchasers. In general, the third-party payers have given inadequate attention to the identification and description of what is being purchased despite extensive efforts to regulate nursing home care. Clearer statements of what the product should be, both in terms of quantity and quality, would in nearly all cases allow more discriminating comparisons of homes and the welfare of patients in various homes, and would force nursing home firms to compete more vigorously.

Strong competition among profit-seeking nursing homes could effectively set the price (and reimbursement rate) for nursing home services. Accordingly, capital owners and workers alike could be paid on the basis of market-determined interest and wage rates.

We know of no careful study comparing a nonregulated competitive nursing home industry with a regulated one. Although certain characteristics of the industry might be difficult to reconcile with a policy of nonregulation, the problems are not trivial, nor are the costs small in establishing and maintaining a comprehensive system of rate setting and regulation in the area of nursing home care. Furthermore, studies that have compared the effects of regulation and nonregulation in other areas have raised substantial doubts about the real advantages of regulation.[5] For these reasons, policymakers should give serious consideration to a policy of nonregulation for the nursing home industry. In any case, the advocates of regulation have a responsibility to demonstrate that the social benefits of regulation are greater than the costs.

The Determination of Market Rents Under Regulation

A cost-related reimbursement and regulatory policy in the nursing home industry can use market incentives to substantial advantage in the payment of capital resources. Capital assets can be viewed as leased by the government for the care of nursing home residents. The issue of reimbursing capital resources then centers on the determination of a rental price. We shall briefly examine the determination of both an explicit and an implicit rental price. Both prices depend upon market activities and can be used to simplify the setting of rents for capital resources in a regulated nursing home industry.

An explicit rental system depends upon a market for leased capital assets. Assets similar to, and in some cases, identical to those in nursing homes are regularly leased. The process is exactly the same as that for labor resources. Rents could be set annually, or as often as necessary, using market surveys, in the same manner as wage levels are determined. In this procedure, the age, condition, location and other characteristics of the assets could be taken into account as are age, education, and experience in the labor force, and a rental price arrived at as a basis for the rent of capital assets used in a nursing home.

Only a relatively small number of services provided in a nursing home are unique (administration of drugs, therapies for disabled residents, and similar medical services); 80–90 percent of the services are comparable to those provided in a hotel, boarding home, or retirement home. The purpose of capital is primarily to produce space. Some equipment is nominally for special purposes in nursing homes, but overall, capital uses compete closely with those in other industries. Furthermore, some nursing home facilities are rented at arm's-length, and these rental agreements provide direct comparisons for assets in nearby and similar nursing homes.

The explicit rental system has two significant advantages. First, the use of market rentals for comparable assets eliminates concern over such questions as who owns what and whether sales are made and to whom. The determination of the market price circumvents most of the reporting, reviewing of records, and auditing concerned with the legitimacy of liabilities, reasonableness of interest payments, amount of and rate of return on equity capital, amount of depreciation, and so forth. Second, the explicit rental payment method is direct and likely to allocate capital most efficiently. What the buyers and sellers of leased assets are willing to pay, or to take, when numerous opportunities are available, is a close approximation of the real productive value of those assets.

This explicit rental system, however, will function well only if there is an effectively organized rental market for assets comparable to those in nursing homes. Such markets are rare. Some metropolitan areas do have them, ranging from hotel space or convalescent and retirement homes to various types of space in apartment buildings, offices, warehouses, and industrial buildings. However, adjusting market rents across assets with different characteristics and uses is a much less understood process than adjusting wages for different workers and occupations. Accordingly, it offers only an imprecise basis for comparison of rents.

In summary, the explicit rental approach does offer a guideline for the reimbursement of capital resources. The use of such a guideline may encourage firms to produce at a level of minimum average costs. The explicit rental approach can also provide capital services consistent with quality care. Furthermore, different types of organizations and capital asset financing and ownership arrangements can exist, grow, or disappear in the midst of competition from all capital asset owners in the market.

In the absence of a well-defined market for leasing nursing home assets, the determination of an implicit rent is another approach to capital reimbursement. This approach minimizes reliance upon historical costs and accounting practices and concentrates on a set of market data which can be combined to determine an implicit rental price. These data, for the most part, must be price indexes or rates set independently of the nursing home industry and applied to market-adjusted asset values in the nursing home.

Assets in a nursing home are broadly classified as land, buildings, and equipment. The latter two depreciate in value, and some allowance must be made in a rental payment for this expense. Furthermore, in each class of asset, ownership is dependent upon the financing arrangement. To simplify these matters, we divide capitial assets into debt capital and equity capital. The "price" for debt capital or equity capital is likely to vary as risk varies between these types. Finally, because a rent is a current market price, the underlying asset values must be current market prices, reflecting adjustment for general inflation and for changes in the relative demand for nursing home capital.

We propose an implicit rental formula for an individual facility below. In this formula, let

R_t = Net annual rent for all capital assets in the nursing home in year t;

HA = Historical cost (purchase price) of depreciable assets in year of purchase a;

kr_t = Remaining life of depreciable assets determined in year t;

k_t = Total life of depreciable assets in year t, where $k_t = kr_t + (t - a)$;

ci_t = Construction cost index in year t, an inflation index for depreciable assets;

CD_t = Current depreciation, $[HA(ci_t/ci_a)] / k_t$, in year t;

CVA_t = Current value of depreciable assets, $CD_t \cdot kr_t$, in year t;

HL = Historical cost (purchase price) of land in year of purchase a;

nd_t = Gross National Product price deflator index in year t, an inflation index for HL;

CVL_t = Current value of land, $HL(nd_t/nd_a)$, in year t;

D_t = Long-term debt in year t (an obligation not due in current fiscal year);

i_t = Market mortgage rate in year t;

E_t = Equity, $CVA_t + CVL_t - D_t$, in year t;

r_t = Market rate of return on equities in year t;

Δ_t = Risk premium, a percentage addition or deduction from the point spread between a "riskless" interest rate and r, in year t.

The *net* rent (exclusive of taxes, insurance, and maintenance costs) would be determined as follows:

$$R_t = \frac{HA\frac{ci_t}{ci_a}}{k_t} + i_t D_t$$

$$+ (r + \Delta)_t \left[\left(\frac{HA\frac{ci_t}{ci_a}}{k_t} \cdot kr_t \right) + HL\frac{nd_t}{nd_a} - D_t \right] \tag{1}$$

or

$$R_t = CD_t + i_t D_t + (r + \Delta)_t (CVA_t + CVL_t - D_t) \tag{2}$$

or

$$R_t = CD_t + i_t D_t + (r + \Delta)_t E_t. \tag{3}$$

The unique aspect of this formula is its use of market data. In all cases the "price" of debt and equity capital is determined explicitly and independently of the nursing home industry. Furthermore, all variables in this rental formula can be determined from directly observable data. Use of the formula minimizes reliance on the subjective judgments of the facility owner/administrator and the regulatory personnel to determine values that will affect property cost reimbursement.

Some data are taken directly from the nursing homes. The historical cost of all assets, including land (HA and HL), and long-term debt (D), are data in the balance sheet of the firm and are easily verifiable from other sources, if necessary. What constitutes long-term debt will require a specific definition, such as an obligation not due in the current fiscal year of the facility. This problem, however, is common to accounting practice and can be resolved.

Information for other variables is easily obtained from sources outside the nursing home. For example, an inflation index for depreciable assets (ci) can be taken from the U.S. Department of Commerce construction cost index for small commercial buildings. Adjusting HA by such an index is essentially a replacement cost strategy commonly used in making property appraisals. Similarly, the GNP price deflator index can be used to adjust land values for inflation, and the rise in the price of land can be approximated.* Further, the interest rate on long-term debt (i) is available from the

---

*Neither the ci nor nd takes account of changes in the relative demand for nursing home services. Because relative demand will change, some adjustments to asset values may have to

Mortgage Bankers Association series on mortgages under $1 million, or from a similar series of lending rates for loans to small businesses comparable to nursing home firms.

The remaining market price is the rate of return for equity capital (r). This rate can be determined from the performance of a "diversified and efficient" portfolio of equity securities on the New York Stock Exchange, or other national stock exchange. We propose that this market rate of return is the one most easily justified under current law and Medicaid regulations as representative of the *cost* of equity funds. However, estimation of risk associated with nursing home investment (Δ) may require either an upward or downward adjustment in the earnings rate of the equities market. Unfortunately, at present there is no commonly accepted method for determining the risk premium for nursing home investment. Research underway at the Battelle Health Care Study Center under the sponsorship of the Health Care Financing Administration promises to be helpful in this regard.[6] The experience of regulated industries would indicate, however, that the risk factor commonly reduces the earning rate to slightly below the equity market rate. A reasonable starting point for cost-based reimbursement regulation would be to take the market rate on equities, r, and in subsequent years to adjust that rate to one comparable with regulated industries. Adjustments might also be made as further research on risk in nursing home investments produces new findings.

The remaining variable to be estimated is the length of life of assets (k). What is allowed for tax purposes by the Internal Revenue Service is one guideline; what experience in the industry has demonstrated is another. Although there appears to be no wide disagreement in the industry on this issue, we suggest that the IRS guidelines for asset life are unrealistic. If we are to follow the market and measure real depreciation in current dollars, then the IRS guidelines for asset life (and particularly for the life of buildings) are too low. These guidelines were established, in part, to encourage investment by allowing book depreciation greater than real depreciation,

---

be made at frequent intervals. Such adjustments would be based on an analysis of such demand factors as the age, income, and geographical distribution of potential users of nursing home services. Another factor which might necessitate changes in asset values would be the growth of the private sector of the industry, including the development of such alternatives to institutional care as domiciliary or home health care.

One further point should be made about the model. Because our intention in designing the model was to demonstrate a particular principle, we have assumed that all assets were purchased at one point in time. Appropriate adjustments could be made by adjusting each asset's purchase price by the appropriate index change since date of purchase. Different inflation indexes could, in fact, be used for different types of assets, such as buildings, equipment, and land.

ceteris paribus. Furthermore, asset durability and length of life are extended by maintenance expenditures, as we pointed out above. Hence, we propose that industry experience is the more reliable guideline at this time. If an implicit rental system is put into effect, a systematic analysis of *actual* length of asset life should be undertaken to determine what guidelines should be used.*

Other elements in the rent formula are computed by use of the variables just discussed. Annual current depreciation (CD) is based on the market value of assets and the expected length of life of the asset. Depreciation is thus measured in current dollars and is not based on the historical cost of the asset. Equity capital (E) is estimated as the difference between the market value of depreciable assets and land and long-term debt. Thus, the equity capital return is in current dollars on the basis of the current value of assets owned.

Consequences of a Rental System

The rental price either explicitly or implicitly determined is a prospective one. The annual rent is set on the basis of values prevailing at the beginning of the year. What happens in the rental, financial, or capital markets during the year, as well as what actions the nursing home administrator takes during the same period, will indeed determine whether the nursing home makes a profit or incurs a loss. But this is as it should be. The owner should be knowledgeable about developments in the market in order to make intelligent decisions and must be given an opportunity to demonstrate a competence that is rewarded by profit, or an inefficiency that results in a loss.

Under a rental system, the owner/investor/administrator is free to arrange ownership of assets in any way; the question of who owns the assets becomes a moot issue in determining the rent for capital assets in a nursing home. Such a system also eliminates much of the costly auditing and monitoring necessary to establish the legitimacy of mortgages, notes, and rental-lease arrangements.

---

*Since kr_t and thus k_t can be changed by the nursing home owner depending on the intensity of use of an asset in relation to the extent of maintenance of the asset and its durability, k cannot be set unequivocally forever at time of purchase. K may also change in reaction to market forces, as do i and r, and thus its value may need to be adjusted periodically in order that the curent depreciation approximates as nearly as possible the real depreciation of the asset. Thus, observation of what actually has occurred in the industry to the lifetime of assets is crucial, and a reassessment of the value attributed to k is important to undertake every few years.

The use of market prices, such as the mortgage interest rate, encourages the nursing home owner to make the most advantageous financing arrangement. If a firm has borrowed at a high interest rate, and the current market mortgage rate falls, the owner has an immediate incentive to refinance: the failure to do so reduces the return on equity capital and may result in losses. If an owner is known to be an efficient manager, lenders may also be willing to provide funds at a lower interest rate than to other borrowers in the current market. The efficient manager will be rewarded under the proposed capital reimbursement plan. The suggested rental system clearly allows the owner/entrepreneur to choose the mix of debt and equity financing preferred and to take into account the risk associated with investment in the nursing home industry and in equity capital, specifically. Further, under either the explicit or implicit rental system, all owners, whether lessors or facility administrators, will receive equal treatment according to the capital resources employed.

A rental system solves some regulatory and capital reimbursement problems, but of course, not all of them. Every reimbursement plan is concerned with the reasonableness of the quantity of capital for each unit of output. For example, how much land, building space, and equipment for each bed would be efficient? This issue is gradually becoming a problem under cost-related reimbursement, especially in the absence of a regulation limiting the per diem reimbursement for "property and related" costs. There is no reason to believe that a rental system approach would aggravate the situation, and, in fact, the opposite may well be the case. Capital reimbursement through either an explicitly or implicitly determined rent has the advantage of identifying more quickly the increasing real rent costs for each patient.*

The merits of a payment system based on market-determined rents are substantial. The rental plan for the reimbursement of capital resources requires serious consideration and may well be a better alternative to current systems of capital reimbursement.

Summary

The reimbursement of capital resources in the determination of a rate for nursing home services in a cost-related reimbursement system has been

---

*The issue here is to avoid the construction of a "marble palace," which would be paid for under any reimbursement plan, if appropriate standards on the quantity of capital are not set. See the discussion of this subject in New York State Moreland Act Commission, pp. 82 ff.

confronted with several problems. First, there are complexities inherent in setting rents on capital resources. These complexities, related to depreciation expense and the return to the services of capital, are not found in the case of wages for labor. Second, regulatory and reimbursement agencies have relied on historical asset costs in determining returns for the services of capital assets. Nursing home owners, however, encouraged by inflation, competition and the normal desire to maximize profits, have made market-oriented adjustments. These adjustments have frequently taken the form of trafficking in nursing homes and sale-lease back arrangements between affiliated organizations. Such practices have resulted from the divergence in market values and historical costs used in state Medicaid reimbursement systems, and are symptomatic of the difficulties in our present reimbursement system.

The problems we have cited suggest that a system that recognizes the real cost of capital services, accounts for risk of investment, and relies more heavily on market forces may be in order. Some evidence indicates that nonregulation may solve more problems and create fewer new ones than a cost-related reimbursement system in the payment for capital services. In the presence of a cost-related system, however, a rental approach for the reimbursement of capital resources would appear to be most advantageous. If markets do not exist where assets are leased and a market rent cannot be determined, an implicit rental system approach is the best solution. This latter approach minimizes reliance upon accounting conventions and historical costs and determines an implicit rent for capital resources on the basis of other sets of related market data.

NOTES

1. New York State Moreland Act Commission on Nursing Homes and Residential Facilities, *Reimbursement of Nursing Home Property Costs: Pruning the Money Tree* (New York: New York State Moreland Act Commission, 1976), pp. 1–177.

2. A detailed discussion of the reasons for differences in book and real rates of return on capital resources is found in Kenneth M. McCaffree, Suresh Malhotra, and John Wills, *Profits, Growth, and Reimbursement Systems in the Nursing Home Industry*, Final Report to the Health Care Financing Administration (Seattle, Washington: Battelle Human Affairs Research Centers). Forthcoming.

3. For a more extended discussion of the definition and role of profit (or loss) see Kenneth M. McCaffree, "Return to Equity Capital in Nursing Homes" (paper presented at the National Long-Term Care Reimbursement Conference, Washington, D.C., February 1976).

4. See Charles L. Schultze, *The Public Use of Private Interest* (Washington, D.C.: The Brookings Institution, 1977).

5. For health care regulation, see Roger G. Noll, "The Consequences of Public Utility Regulation of Hospitals," in National Academy of Sciences, Institute of Medicine, *Controls on Health Care* (Washington, D.C.: National Academy of Sciences, 1975), pp. 25–48; and U.S., Department of Health, Education, and Welfare, Public Health Service, National Center

for Health Services Research, "Impact of State Certificate of Need Laws on Health Care Costs and Utilization," *Research Digest Series*, by David S. Salkever and Thomas W. Bice, DHEW Pubn. No. (HRA) 77-3163 (Washington, D.C., 1977). For a general critique of regulation and supporting references, see Schultze, *Public Use*.

6. McCaffree et al., *Profits, Growth, and Reimbursement Systems*. This is a further extension of work on the capital asset pricing model begun by the Battelle group in 1974. See Kenneth M. McCaffree, Kavasseri V. Ramanathan, Lawrence D. Muller, Michael Maher, and L. Charles Miller, Jr., *Profit and Growth: Allowances for Owner/Operator Contributions in a Cost-Related Prospective Payment for Services System for Nursing Home Care* (Washington, D.C.: American Health Care Association, 1975).

INDEX

accreditation, regulation and, 91–92, 100–01, 102–03
Administration on Aging, 18, 58
Administrative Procedures Act, 172
aged, 8, 17, 81, 113, 173; in community, 17–19; costs of illness, average out-of-pocket, 27; day care, 38; frail elderly, 19; home health care, 37–38; impairments, chronic, 19–20; in institutions, 19–21; integration of services for, 52; mentally impaired, 24, 42; in psychiatric facilities, 25; services received by, 20–25
Alabama, 42
Altman, Stuart, 88, 89
Ambulatory Chronic Care Service Proposal, 5, 55–56; federal role, 59–60; financing, 57, 59; housing programs, 58–59; populations, eligible, 57; program structure, 56–61; service structure, 57–58; social services, 58; state role, 60; Supplemental Security Income, 59
American Association of Homes for the Aging, 118
American Health Care Association, 118
American Hospital Association, 88
American Institute of Certified Public Accountants, 130–31
American Medical Association, 88
Arthur Bolton Associates, 25
Arthur D. Little, Inc., 90
assessment-coordination system: function of, 30–31; models, 31–33; need, 29–30
audits and audit agencies, 4, 7, 126–52; audit universe, 128; comprehensive program, state level, 7; coordination of and cooperation in, 11; definition of audit, 128; duplication of coverage, 143; follow-up, 7, 148–50; guidelines and standards, 128–31; evaluations and audits, 150–51; federal vs. state interests, 147; multiple agency system, 7; performance audits, 7, 148; problems, financial and operational, 142–51; procedures, overview of current, 127–42; program management and, 7, 151; and regulation, 7, 11;

reimbursement of costs of, 144–46; single-audit concept, 143–44; state, 7, 128, 133–34, 138–41 (*see also* names of agencies)

Baldwin, John R., 85
Ball, Robert, 87
Battelle Health Care Study Center, 206
Bauer, Katherine, 90
Bernstein, Marver H., 85, 86, 102
Berry, Ralph E., 89
Bice, Thomas W., 91
Blue Cross, 90
boarding homes, 39, 43
budgets vs. insurance financing, 71–72

California, 36, 68–69, 146
capital expenditures, regulation of, 90–91
Carmel, Harvey, 9, 176–86
certification, regulation and, 91–92, 100–01, 102–03
children, mentally retarded or physically disabled, 22
Clark, Arva, 90
Code of Federal Regulations, 94
community care services, 11; and aged, 17–19; and Ambulatory Chronic Care Service proposal, 61; appropriateness of placement in, 33–36; assessment-coordination system, models for, 31–33; costs, 36; developments in, 36–40; expansion of, 11, 12–14; federal grants to as option, 73–74; financing as spur to development, 10–11, 60; and institutional placement, 33–44; and Medicaid, 45–46; for mentally ill or retarded, 23, 26, 43; support services, 38–40 (*see also* specific services)
Community Mental Health Centers, 23, 26, 43, 50; Act of 1973, 50
Community Services Administration, 131
congregate care, 6
continuity of services, 11
contracts, service, 33
coordination of care, 12; assessment and, 29–33; Ambulatory Chronic Care Service proposal, 5, 55–61; components of system of, 26–33; frag-

211

mentation of service efforts, 52–53; "level of care" barriers to, 53–54; management and treatment patterns, 26–28; methods of, 31–33; and public programs, 52–55; purpose and functions, 30–31

Correia, Eddie W., 5–6, 9, 10–11, 65–80

costs, 27, 69; audit, reimbursement of, 144–46; capital resources, and reimbursement, 187–209; depreciation, 187, 189, 192–93, 195–96; dietary services, 9; engineering model for determination of, 8, 263–65; homemaker service, 70; hospital, 88–90; nursing, 9; nursing homes, 9, 177–209; operating, of nursing home, 177–78; regulation and, 3, 9, 88–90, 109–10, 175, 176–86, 187–209; reimbursement policy and, 89–90; sharing, by patient, 10, 75; statistical model for determination of, 8, 157–63 (*see also* financing)

counseling, 11

courts: and mentally impaired, 42; role of, 4

data collection systems, 9

day care, 6, 11, 38; and Medicaid, 46; of mentally retarded, 23

definition of long-term care, 16, 65

deinstitutionalization, 12–15, 40; of mentally retarded or ill, 23, 25, 41–42, 43, 108

developmentally disabled, 22, 50–51

Dias, Robert M., 7, 11, 126–52

dietary services, 9

disabled, 8; definition of, 1–2; physically disabled adults, 21–22; services for, 2; and Title XX of Social Security Act, 49; veterans, 2

discontinuity, program, 11

District of Columbia, 90–91

Economic Stabilization Program, 88–89

Eichenholz, Joseph, 88, 89

eligibility criteria, 2–3, 4, 68, 75

Environmental Protection Agency, 146

evaluation: audits and, 150–51; and diagnosis, in assessments-coordination system of services, 30–31

Federal Council on Aging, 19

federal government and programs, 6, 44–55; and Ambulatory Chronic Care Service proposal, 59–60; coordination

barriers, 52–55; financing by, 5–6, 35, 44–52, 65–80 (*see also* specific programs and subjects); regulatory policies, 6–7; vocational rehabilitation, 2 (*see also* specific subjects)

Federal Housing Administration, 169

Federal Management Circulars: No. 73-2, 145, 146; No. 74-4, 145, 146

financing, 4, 5–6, 65–80; Ambulatory Chronic Care Service proposal, 57, 59; by cash payments based on disability of recipient, 72; and coordination of services, 29–30; cost-sharing, patient, 70, 75; costs of proposed model, 76–77; by grants to local agencies, 73–74; by grants to states on income and population basis, 73, 74; insurance vs. fixed budgets, 71–72; by insurance-vendor payments system, 72, 74; matching funds, 10, 35, 73, 74–78, 113; model proposed, 74–79; non-institutional care, incentive for, 10–11, 60; options, 72–74; placement appropriateness and, 35; planning, issues in, 69–72 (*see also* Medicaid; Medicare; reimbursement; etc.)

Florida, 34

follow-up: in assessment-coordination system, 31; of audits, 7, 148–50

foster care, 39; of mentally ill or retarded, 23, 25, 42

General Accounting Office, 11, 127–28, 131, 136–38, 144, 145

General Services Administration Circular No. 73-2, 143

Georgia, 98

Ginsburg, Paul, 89

Great Britain, 38

group homes, 39–40 (*see also* halfway houses)

growth of long-term care, 167–74

halfway houses, 39; for mentally ill or retarded, 23, 25, 42

handicapped (*see* disabled)

Havighurst, Clark C., 91

Health Care Financing Administration, 83, 94

Health, Education, and Welfare, Department of, 54, 83, 89; Audit Agency, 11, 127, 128, 131–36, 144, 148–51; audits of programs of, 136–35; Office of Investigations and Security, 132;

placement, appropriateness of, 3, 33–36, 68, 98; deinstitutionalization and, 42–43

planning, 60; assessment and, 32–33; and ·insurance vs. budget allocation, 71–72; resource allocation, 69–70; states and latitude in use of federal funds, 70–71

populations, long-term care, 17, 18, 65; aged, 17–21; and Ambulatory Chronic Care Service proposal, 57; definition of, 1–2; mentally ill, 24–26; mentally retarded and developmentally disabled, 22–23; noninstitutionalized, 17–19, 67; physically disabled adult, 21–22; services for, 2, 4, 5, 28–29; (*see also* specific subjects)

Posner, Richard A., 85

Professional Standards Review Organizations, 92–93

protective living settings: psychiatric, 25–26; support services, 38–40

psychiatric facilities: and deinstitutionalization, 42–43; inpatient care, 24–25; Medicaid and, 45; readmissions, 43; outpatient services, 23, 25, 26

Public Law 92-603, 54–55, 89, 90, 92–93, 114, 171, 187, 195

Public Law 93-641, 90, 108–09, 111–12, 114

rates, setting of, 11; and capital reimbursement, 189–91; and regulation, 93, 109

reform, perspectives on, 3–12; and implementation problems, 12–15

regulation, 2–3, 4, 6, 8, 41, 81–125; in acute health care sector, 87–93; audits and, 7,11; bed supply and, 102–03; of capital expenditures, 90–91; certificate-of-need process, 90–91, 112, 113, 191; coordination of, 11; cost controls, 88–90, 109–10; costs for, 3, 9, 175, 176–86; environment of, improving the, 112–17, 174–75; failures of, 97–103; history, brief, 83–84; implementation of reform of, 117–19; inspection process and, 99–101, 107–08, 111–12; legal process and, 101; licensure, certification, and accreditation, 91–92, 96, 100–01, 102–03, 107, 114; "lifecycle" schema of, 86, 102; limitations on effectiveness of, 99–103; in long-term health care sector, 86–87, 93–119; by market, 85, 87, 104–06; market rental determination under, 202–08,

Medicaid/Medicare and, 41, 93–98, 112–17 *passim* ; in other sectors of economy, 84–87; peer review and, 92–93; policy options, 103–07; politics and, 101–02; process improvement, 107–12; public utility approach, 84, 93, 105; and quality of care, 88–89, 92, 93, 109, 113–14; rate setting and, 93, 109; reimbursement policy and, 9, 89–90, 109–10, 112–13; requirements, streamlining, 110–11; responsibility and, 102–03, 107–09; theories of, 84–87; and "trafficking" in nursing homes, 191–92, 196–200

rehabilitative services: audits of, 129, 132; under Medicaid, 45; under Medicare, 47; veterans, 51; vocational, 2, 50

reimbursement: Ambulatory Chronic Care Service proposal, 60; of audit costs, 144–46; of capital expenditures, 90–91; for capital investment and service, 187–209; and cost containment, 89–90; cost-related, 7–8, 112, 157–63, 187, 195–96; in Illinois, 154–56, 157; market rental system, for capital resources, 202–08; by Medicaid, 10, 35, 45–46, 52–55, 69, 89, 93–94, 112, 113, 196–98; by Medicare, 90–91, 93–94, 112, 113; nonregulated, of capital resources, 201–02; patient health status index and, 6, 110; patient-related, 153–67; and placement appropriateness, 35; point count system of, 154–56; problems of, 8; quality of care and, 6, 10; regulatory policy and, 9, 109–10, 112–13; Supplemental Security Income and, 54–55

representation and mediation, in assessment-coordination sysem of services, 31

research programs, 116–17

residential facilities, small, 3

Rhode Island, 97, 98, 101, 103

Roemer, Milton I., 92

Ruchlin, Hirsch S., 6, 9, 10, 11, 81–125

Rush-Presbyterian-St. Luke's Medical Center (Chicago), 116

Salkever, David W., 91

Services Integration for Deinstitutionalization Project, 30

services, long-term care, 2, 4, 15, 28–29; Ambulatory Chronic Care Service proposal, 57–59; assessment-coordi-

215

ABOUT THE AUTHORS

VALERIE LaPORTE is chief editorial associate in the Disability and Health Economics Research Section of the Bureau of Economic Research at Rutgers University. She has assisted in editing several volumes in the areas of public policy and health, including *An Evaluation of Policy-Related Rehabilitation Research* (New York: Praeger Publishers, 1975) and *Public Policy Toward Disability* (New York: Praeger Publishers, 1976).

JEFFREY RUBIN is an assistant professor of economics at Rutgers and assistant director of the Disability and Health Economics Research Section of the Bureau of Economic Research. He is the author of 2Economics, Mental Health and the Law (Lexington, Mass.: D. C. Heath, Lexington Books, 1978), and co-author of *An Evaluation of Policy-Related Rehabilitation Research* (New York: Praeger Publishers, 1975).

HARVEY CARMEL is currently a private consultant in health planning. He has held the position of Deputy Director of the Health Education Council in Baltimore. His professional activities include the design of programs to implement shared service arrangements between hospitals and long-term care providers.

EDDIE W. CORREIA is an attorney in the Cleveland Regional Office of the Federal Trade Commission. He has worked as a consultant to the Office of the Assistant Secretary for Planning and Evaluation in the Department of Health, Education, and Welfare. His articles have appeared in *The American Journal of Public Health* and the *Oklahoma Law Review*.

ROBERT M. DIAS is a CPA who is currently a consultant in private practice. He has served as an audit manager for the Department of Health, Education, and Welfare. He is the author of a number of texts on accounting, auditing, and quantitative methods.

JUDITH LaVOR heads the Long Term Care Coverage Branch, Office of Demonstrations and Evaluations in the Health Care Financing Administration of the Department of Health, Education, and Welfare. Her previous experience includes work in the Office of the Assistant Secretary for Planning and Evaluation and in the Office of Nursing Home Affairs. She has written extensively on long-term care policy and the feasibility of home health care as an alternative to institutionalization.

SURESH MALHOTRA is a research scientist at the Battelle Human Affairs Centers. He has conducted research on the impact of unemployment on the health insurance coverage of workers and is currently investigating the effects of state Medicaid reimbursement systems on the growth of the nursing home industry.

KENNETH M. McCAFFREE is a research scientist at the Battelle Human Affairs Research Centers in Seattle. He is also a professor of economics and professor of health services at the University of Washington. His articles on nursing homes have appeared in the *American Health Care Association Journal* and the *Gerontologist*.

HIRSCH S. RUCHLIN is professor of economics in public health at the Cornell University Medical College. His articles on long term care have appeared in the *Journal of Health Politics, Policy and Law, Topics in Health Care Financing, Medical Care*, and the *Americal Journal of Public Health*. He is also the co-author of *Economics and Health Care* (Springfield, Ill.: Charles C. Thomas, 1973).

THOMAS J. WALSH is the associate director for Health Finance in the Illinois Department of Public Health. He has served as a consultant to the Health Care Financing Administration, the Center for Health Services Research and Development, and the Bureau of Health Planning Research and Development. He has also written several articles on state and local finance issues.

HARVEY WERTLIEB is the owner-administrator of the Randolph Hills Nursing Home in Maryland. He has been an associate professorial lecturer at George Washington University and has served as a member of the editorial board of *Long Term Care Administration*. He is currently Executive Editor of *Nursing Homes*.

JOHN WILLS is a research scientist at the Battelle Human Affairs Centers. He has undertaken studies of the determinants of job-related health insurance coverage and the effect of reimbursement policy on nursing home rates of return. He is the editor of ''Proceedings of a Conference on Model Validation,'' which documented a 1977 forum sponsored by the National Bureau of Economic Research.